Franklin H. Martin, MD, FACS:

From Rural Boyhood to Distinguished Surgeon

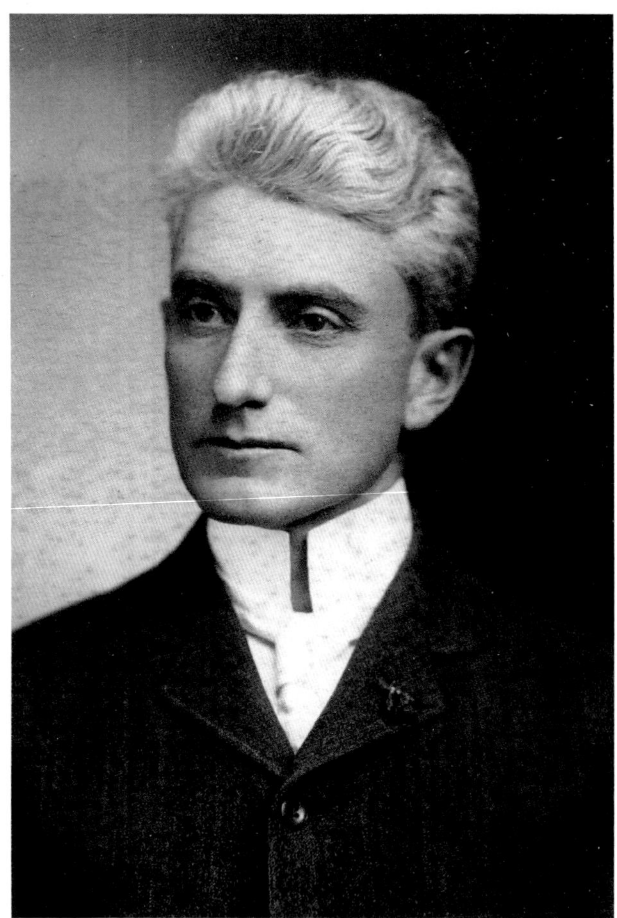

Franklin H. Martin, MD, FACS, founder of the American College of Surgeons, circa 1900.

Franklin H. Martin, MD, FACS:
From Rural Boyhood to Distinguished Surgeon

Gordon L. Telford, MD, FACS

American College of Surgeons • Chicago, IL

ISBN: 978-1-7337149-9-0

Front cover photos, insets: Franklin Martin, circa the time he left for medical school in Chicago and in the early 1930s. Background: The field where Franklin was binding oats when he saw Dr. Daniel McLaren Miller drive by in his buggy and decided to become a doctor (photo by Gordon L. Telford).

Book design by Tina Woelke

American College of Surgeons
633 N. Saint Clair Street
Chicago, IL 60611-3295

www.facs.org

Printed in the United States of America

Dedication

To my wife Susan and my daughter Elizabeth
for their constant support and assistance
and in loving memory of my son Andy
this book is dedicated.

Table of Contents

Preface

Many years ago, at the annual Clinical Congress of the American College of Surgeons (ACS), I spoke with Susan Rishworth, who was then the ACS Archivist. In the course of our conversation, she became aware that I lived in the same area of southern Wisconsin where Franklin H. Martin, founder of the ACS, was born and lived for the first 20 years of his life. We discussed the fact that the College had minimal detailed information about where Martin was born and the areas where he lived, attended school, played, worked, and matured into a young man. We discussed my taking on the project of researching in detail his early life in Wisconsin, and she was incredibly supportive of my doing just that. I agreed that it sounded like an exciting and interesting project and one that I would enjoy performing. Little did I know at that time how many years I would spend on the research and how much could be learned about Martin's character by exploring his early life.

When I began this endeavor, my main objective was simply to document Martin's early years, but as I progressed it became obvious that his rural upbringing had a tremendous impact on his character and fostered attributes that made it feasible for him to accomplish all he did in his lifetime. It then became important to me that I write this book and elaborate on the characteristics that resulted from his rural upbringing and the impact they had on his career and life.

Because his autobiography, *The Joy of Living*, is essentially the only source for firsthand information about Martin's early life, I have liberally used the book to inform the chapters covering his life up to age 20. I also had access to Martin's handwritten first draft of volume one of his autobiography, which is in the Martin Collection of the Archives of the American College of Surgeons. The majority was composed on hotel stationery. Surprising, large parts of his first draft were minimally changed in the published book. The draft was fascinating to read and offered further insight into his life. *The Joy of Living* contains vast amounts of general information, but it is lacking in specifics, which made the initial work slow going. For instance, Martin listed the location of the family farms as being at the "big bend" in the Rock River. Next question: which big bend in the Rock River? I visited the Jefferson County Courthouse and the Dodge/Jefferson County Historical Society Library, where I found a plat map from 1862 with the locations of Martin's mother's and father's family homesteads. State, county, and local historical societies can be helpful in conducting this type of historical research. Not only do they have large collections of documents, often they have enthusiastic members who love to help amateur historical researchers like me. City libraries also may have large collections of historical materials. It is sometimes necessary to consult all these sources when attempting to verify information.

Other effective sources were the centennial and sesquicentennial books written by residents of small towns. An example of such a book is *Heritage of Ixonia* by Alida and Carl Jaeger, written in celebration of Ixonia's sesquicentennial. Searching the archives of local newspapers also was useful. Of course, many of the sources I mention now are available online, making this type of research much easier.

One of the most important aspects of historical research is browsing archival materials. Besides being a necessary research tool, it can be enjoyable and lead to new insights. As I proceeded with my research, it became obvious that other surgeons from Martin's and later eras believed they had benefited from a rural upbringing, which strengthened my hypothesis.

My experience tells me that you either enjoy this type of research or you don't; there doesn't appear to be much middle ground. Just like other types of research, such as genealogy, research into a historical topic can take many years. You must be happy if you establish one new fact after a day of work—such as where the "big bend" in the Rock River is located. This project was full of such moments of discovery.

Gordon L. Telford, MD, FACS

Introduction

Franklin H. Martin spent most of the first 20 years of his life in rural Wisconsin. His was a rather typical rural upbringing. At age nine he was working on his grandfather's farm, helping plant and harvest crops and caring for the animals. For the next 11 years, he worked as a farm laborer, brickmaker, janitor, schoolteacher, and millwright. He left Wisconsin at age 20 to attend Chicago Medical School from 1877 to 1880. He then completed a one-year internship at Mercy Hospital in Chicago, something that only a few medical school graduates did at that time. In 1881, he began practicing obstetrics and gynecology in Chicago.

During all phases of his long career, Martin was an uncommonly accomplished physician, administrator, and leader—admired and arguably emulated by his peers as well as by those younger and less experienced. It is my assertion that it wasn't in spite of his rural upbringing in Wisconsin that he became a great leader—it was because of it.

Because of the values his family had imbued in him, Martin had the strength of character, the self-confidence, and the ability to proceed when others might have wavered. Those values came to the fore when he was a child working with his Grandfather Carlin and were reinforced when he worked in the fields and in the brickyard with his cousins and uncles, who taught him the value of hard work and tenacity. He stood side by side with them in the fields—in the sweltering sun and in the pouring rain. He, like his family members, worked to the point of exhaustion. Years later, as an administrator, no matter how stressful his workday was, he recalled that the days in the fields and brickyard were much more exhausting and stressful. Martin learned that hard work yielded results, and he never lost that drive.

A significant example of his ability to push forward when others might waver was in 1888, when at age 31 he cofounded the Post-Graduate Medical School and Hospital of Chicago. He was the principal force in organizing the school, with its distinguished teaching faculty and its onsite hospital and clinics. The school offered doctors the opportunity to learn the evaluation, diagnosis, and treatment of clinical entities unfamiliar to them in an era when medical knowledge was rapidly expanding. The school was a successful endeavor that Martin took from conception to functioning entity in seven months, demonstrating the exceptional organizational skills that were going to shape his career and his many accomplishments. Other examples of his organizational skills were his founding of the journal *Surgery, Gynecology and Obstetrics* in 1905, his founding of the Clinical Congress of the Surgeons of North America in 1910, and his founding of the American College of Surgeons in 1913.

Martin never clearly stated where the title for his autobiography—*The Joy of Living*—came from and why he chose it. He used the phrase "joy of living" three times in the book. Once was in reference to how he felt his cousins lived their lives: "...to enjoy life in an environment of honest, God-fearing people who were full of the joy of living."[1] Martin believed that work was a necessity to them, and in their eyes no man was meaner than he who shirked his daily task. Theirs was an outdoor life, and they never tired of hard work. Most of their recreational activities also were centered on the wonderful environment in which they lived. Martin both admired and envied their lifestyle, and in my mind that is why he titled his autobiography *The Joy of Living.*

Another time he used the phrase was about the new life that he was looking forward to living with the start of medical school in Chicago: "Our young souls were filled with joy; and this joy of living was enhanced by anticipation of the immediate future."[2] Most certainly, he anticipated that his new life would give him the same joy that his cousins experienced on the farm.

Lastly, he used the phrase when comparing his and Isabelle's experience attending Chicago Cubs' baseball games and his experience working in Wisconsin in his youth: "...an intangible something brought health, extreme joy of living, and 'pep' that I had not enjoyed since my labors in the brickyard or on the farm."[3] Once again, we see that he first experienced the joy of living while working outdoors during his early years in Wisconsin.[3]

George W. Crile, MD, FACS, said of Martin's early life,

> ...he fought, and played, and sang, and loved; he tested the life of the farmer's chore boy; he made bricks; he was an amateur carpenter; he taught school. By nature sensitive, shy, resourceful, tenacious, with a vivid imagination, with faith and courage, this product of the covered wagon found his way out of the heat and barbs of the harvest field as the result of the lure of medicine, which, too, was in the covered wagon stage. As a student, young Martin won distinction which placed his ambitious foot on the first round of the ladder.[4]

REFERENCES

1. Martin, F. H. (1933). *The Joy of Living: An Autobiography*, vol. 1 (p. 149). New York, NY: Doubleday, Doran & Co.
2. Ibid., p. 128.
3. Ibid., p. 318.
4. Crile, G. Foreword. In: Martin, F. H. (1933). *The Joy of Living: An Autobiography*, vol. 1 (p. xiii). New York, NY: Doubleday, Doran & Co.

Chapter 1

Family Background

~~~ noised ab ~~~
that the Corliss those ~~ ~~ thought
session on Sunday had ~~~
claim on the big bend. Every ~~~
the raising on Saturday. Volunteers
~~hands~~ were busy from all the neig
the week, felling trees, hewing ~~the~~ and adding
the shape for the new house. Early
g of Saturday a dozen or more ~~~
and boys were on hand to construct
house. ~~A~~ cellar had been dug in
~~~ ready to be encased with ~~~
~~~ logs had been sunk in ~~~
reached a bed of solid clay beneath
~~~, lumber had been brought from
~~~ mill and a fine lot of dry ~~~
been contributed by generous neighbors
~~~ ~~oxen~~ ready to compete with ~~~
~~~ sturdy oxen that had been brought
neighbors.

Tom Mortin by common ~~~
~~~ for the day. No time was
of the game
all devotions came the great logs
~~~ chains about their necks ~~~
~~~ of the faithful oxen ~~~

The Carlins and Martins Migrate to Wisconsin

Franklin Martin's parents, Edmond Martin and Josephine Carlin, met in rural Wisconsin when their families settled there in the late 1840s. In June 1847, 13-year-old Edmond Martin (Figure 1.1) left Ontario, Canada, with his parents, William and Caroline Martin (Figure 1.2), and his eight siblings, ranging in age from eight to 28, in search of a new home in the U.S. The Martins traveled west in a large, sturdy oxen-drawn covered wagon. They sold most of their belongings before leaving Canada and converted them to gold. The family began the trek westward with William leading the oxen and Caroline, her family Bible at her feet, sitting in the front of the wagon. The younger children were stowed in the back of the wagon while the older boys walked along behind leading the animals, including a young steer to butcher for sustenance if their hunting failed to produce adequate food. They were uncertain where they would settle, but knew it had to be far enough west that they could buy a farm with the amount of gold they had in their possession. The Martins hoped to settle in Wisconsin, where the broad rivers, numerous lakes, and tall maple trees were reminiscent of their Canadian home.

After leaving Canada, the family stopped in Oswego, NY, for a few months to rest. They slowly continued their trek west through Pennsylvania, Ohio, Indiana, and Illinois, and eventually arrived in Wisconsin. They passed through Milwaukee and came to the beautiful lake region where they hoped to settle. Regrettably, the more desirable homesites near the lakes and streams had already been purchased. But just west of this area they were able to purchase a 100-acre tract of land in Ixonia on the Rock River, 35 miles west of Milwaukee, and built their first home. As described by Martin, "The tract was framed by giant elms, mossy green banks, and surrounding groves of trees—hard maple, butternut, walnut, and ash."[1]

Using the Ancestry.com database, I was able to establish that the Martins were an old New England family. Franklin Martin's ances-

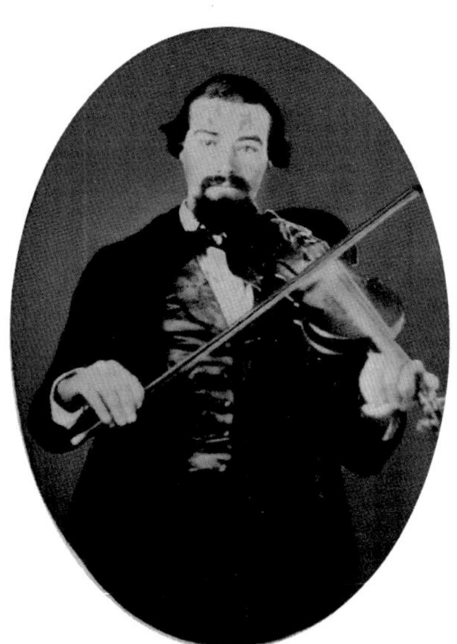

1.1. Edmond Martin, Franklin's father.

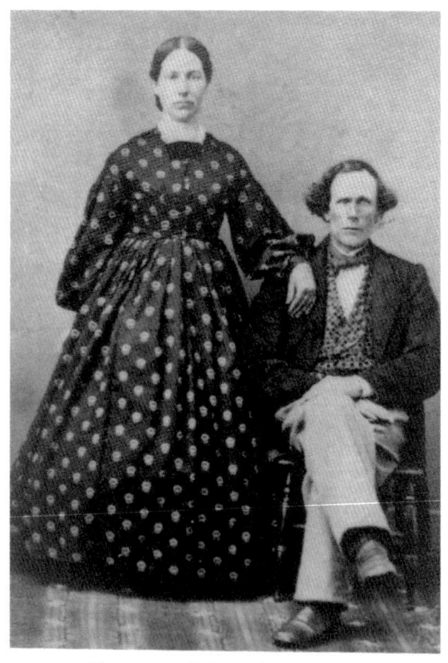

1.2. William and Caroline (Phelps) Martin, Franklin's paternal grandparents.

tor, George Martin, likely emigrated from Hampshire, England, to Massachusetts in approximately 1640, and the family remained there until William and Caroline Martin moved to Canada in approximately 1820. Dr. Martin believed that his paternal ancestors were of Germanic origin, but this supposition likely was incorrect; they were probably British.

In 1849, 11-year-old Josephine Carlin (Figure 1.3) traveled to Wisconsin from Erie County, PA, with her parents, Alexander and Ella Carlin, and her five siblings. Initially the conservative Ella was unwilling to move out west, but eventually Alexander convinced her. The most problematic decision for the family was whether to use their prized white horses to pull their wagon or trade them "for a yoke of strong oxen." Alexander and the children wanted to keep their "pet horses," while Ella felt that oxen would serve them better on the trek west and when they made ready their new farm. Eventually Alexander and the children won out. The Carlins' horse-drawn wagon made the westward trek faster than the Martin family's oxen-drawn wagon had done two years

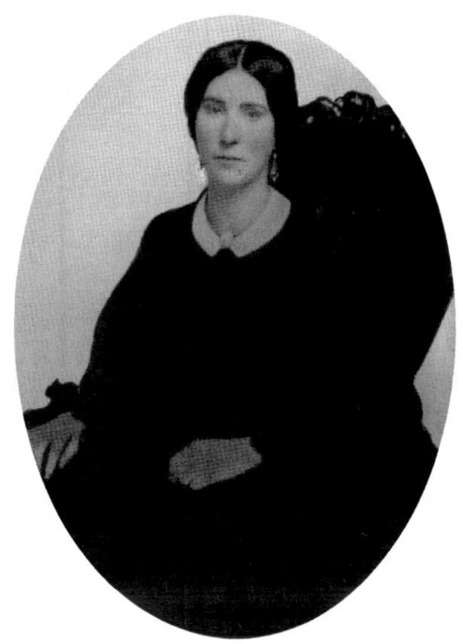

1.3. Josephine Carlin Martin, Franklin's mother.

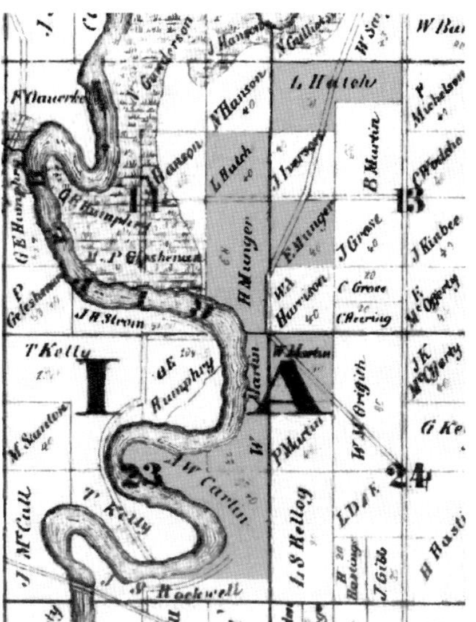

1.4. 1862 plat map of Ixonia Township showing the location of the Martin and Carlin homesteads and the location of Martin's Uncle Luther Hatch's and his stepfather Elon Munger's family homesteads.

before. Addison, the eldest son, had purchased a new pony and it joined the other animals following behind the wagon. The pony brought much pleasure to the family on the trip west. On many days, one of the girls rode the pony, lessening the crowding in the wagon. After a two-month trek, they, too, arrived in the lake country, but found they could not afford property there, primarily because the less-expensive government land had been claimed. As they continued west, they also came upon the wide, deep Rock River, where they set up camp. Everyone, including the horses, enthusiastically embraced their new surroundings. The Carlins knew immediately that this was where they wanted to settle.

As they surveyed the river north and south, their enthusiasm only increased. When they regrouped for supper, the children reported that the swimming was glorious, and the fish and game were plentiful. The following day they continued to explore the river and the surrounding countryside. As described by Martin, "Half a mile to the north the bank was higher, with a mossy slope to the water's edge, and the river bent abruptly to the west. A great forest of hard maples spread away to the north and to the east."[2] Their spirits waned when they met a man who had staked a claim on the land the Carlins desired. Alexander was non-committal when the man asked about their plans. The man offered up that the women of his family were unhappy living in this isolated area. By chance, the Carlins met the Martins, who invited them to dinner. It was Sunday and the Martins were having, as was usual with them, a large meal with their extended family. Before dinner young Edmond Martin took Josephine and Mary Carlin for a river ride in his self-made dugout canoe.[2]

It was the beginning of a warm friendship between Edmond and Josephine. At dinner there were introductions all around. Three of the Martin girls had married local men, as frequently happened in the 1800s when young people were seldom able to travel far from home to meet suitable partners. Ten of the Carlin and Martin offspring present at the dinner either were married to or would marry someone who lived within two to three miles of the homesteads. Lucretia Martin was married to William Fulmer, and Betsy Martin to William's brother George. Melissa Martin was with her husband James Padden. The young Martins—Phineas, Edmond, Richard, Terressa, Millie (Permelia), and Jane—also were in attendance, along with the young Carlins—Addison, Mary, Josephine, Henry, and Henderson.[3]

While walking back to their camp, Alexander Carlin had an opportunity to talk to the man who owned the parcel of land next to the Martin's homestead, and he offered to purchase the land. Much to his surprise, the next morning the landowner agreed to sell (Figure 1.4). Regrettably, Alexander did not obtain a proper survey, which later led to a major disagreement between the Carlins and Martins. Within the week a house-raising was arranged and the neighbors were invited to help. By the end of the day, the basic structure was completed, and the Carlins had a home.[4]

Again, using Ancestry.com, I was able to confirm that Alexander Carlin's grandfather, Franklin's great-great-grandfather, had emigrated to Pennsylvania from Ireland in the mid-eighteenth century, as Franklin noted in his autobiography. Not much else is known about his Carlin ancestors.

The Carlin family home (Figure 1.5) and the Martin family home (Figure 1.6) are still on the homestead land. Upon arriving in the area, both families realized that the surroundings, with a broad deep river,

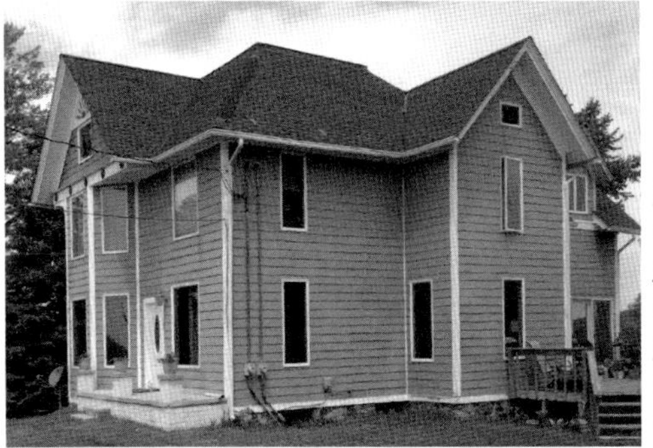

1.5. Recent photograph of the Carlin family's home in Ixonia Township. The site of this home agrees with the site identified on plat maps from the mid-1800s. In addition, close examination of the foundation of the home reveals that it was constructed with fieldstone, making it likely that the home was built in the mid-1800s, when the Carlins lived there.

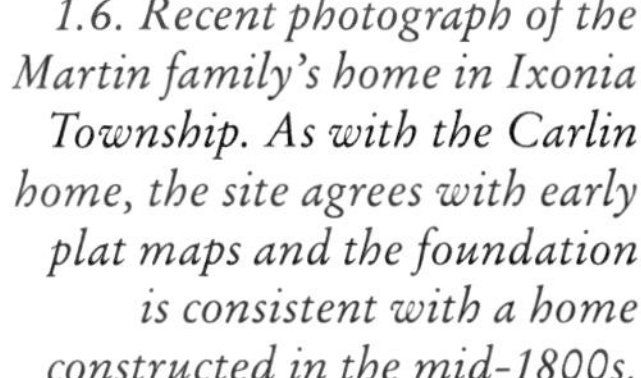

1.6. Recent photograph of the Martin family's home in Ixonia Township. As with the Carlin home, the site agrees with early plat maps and the foundation is consistent with a home constructed in the mid-1800s.

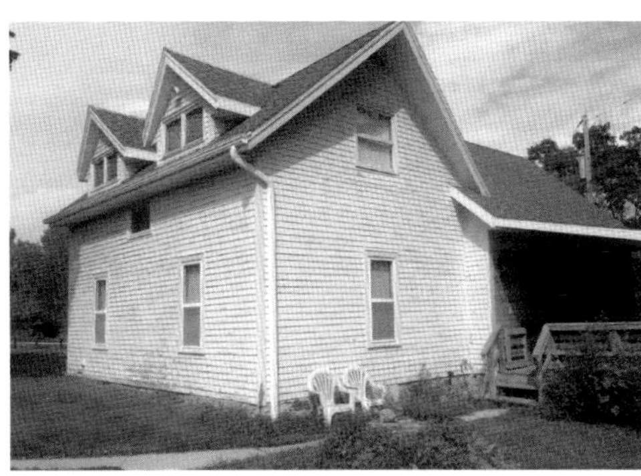

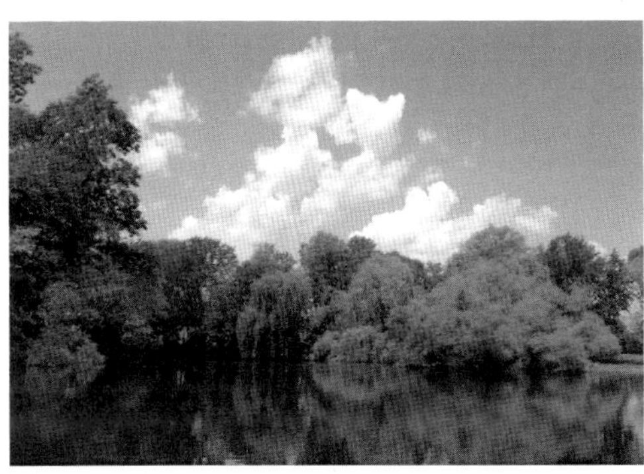

1.7a. Recent photograph of the area where the Martins and Carlins homesteaded on the Rock River, showing what a beautiful area it is.

1.7b. Martin's 1918 photograph of the same area.

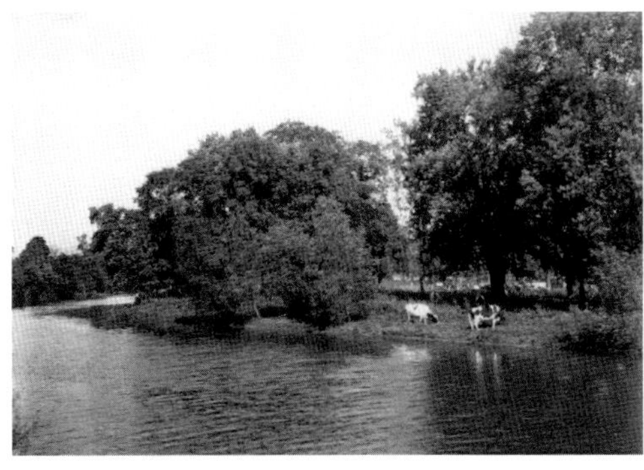

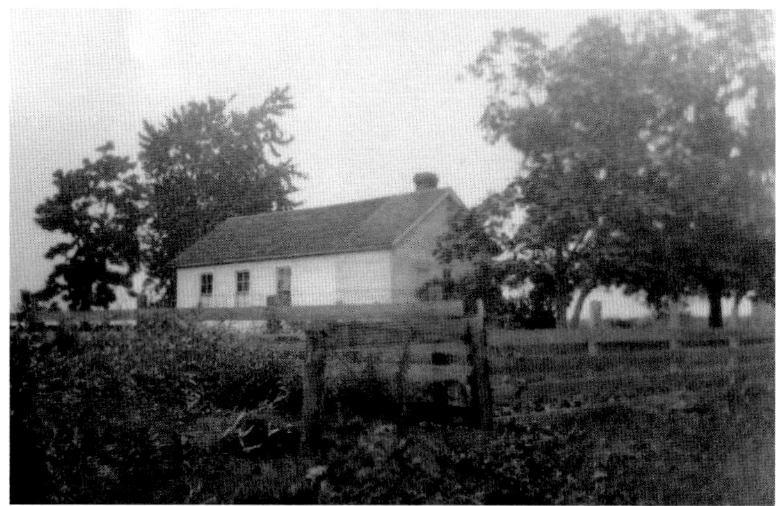

1.8. Franklin's parents' home on the Martin homestead land, where Martin lived up to age 10.

fertile soil, and tall hardwood trees, would be an enjoyable place to live. In Martin's words, "Even the tired horses pricked their ears and sniffed of the fresh air."[5] The area is still lush today, and it is obvious why they would have desired settling there (Figures 1.7a and 1.7b).[5]

Parents' Courtship and Marriage

Over the next five years, Edmond and Josephine became companions and good friends. As their friendship grew, Edmond was becoming a respected carpenter, known for his substantial and durable work. His workshop, which he had built to accommodate his ever-enlarging woodworking business, had two large rooms, one for storage and the other for his work. It was a solidly constructed building framed with timbers, covered with clapboards, and had a well-shingled roof. It was a gathering place for family and friends. As Josephine matured into a young woman, Edmond began to court her. They were married June 24, 1856, and moved into Edmond's shop, which he had converted into a small home.[6]

On July 13, 1857, Franklin Martin was born in his parents' two-room home on the banks of the Rock River (Figure 1.8). Franklin's mother Josephine was 19 years old and his father Edmond 23 years old.[7]

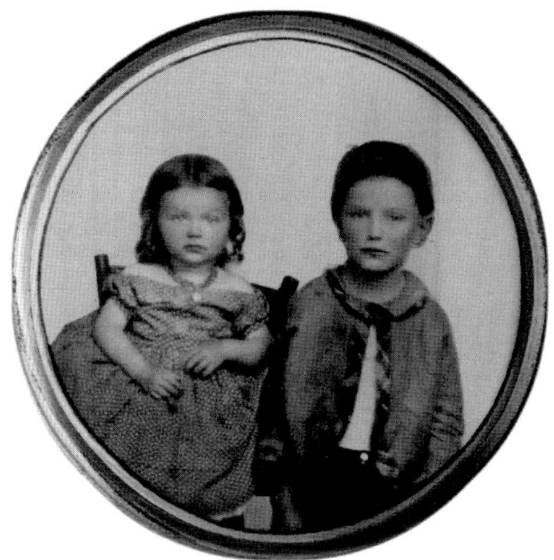

1.9. Franklin and his sister Jeanette at a young age.

The Extended Family

In his autobiography, Martin describes the Martins and Carlins as "tillers of the soil, and had little thought but to live respectable lives and earn their bread by the sweat of their brows" and "They were of sound stock. They possessed sane minds. They were temperate in eating and drinking." They were religious but, except for Grandmother Caroline Martin, did not attend church. Franklin Martin later said that they were honest, not scandalous, and patriotic, law-abiding citizens. He described them as "uneducated in the modern sense of the term, but well grounded" in the basics, and they were the kind of people who "formed the backbone of our country." In his words, "Their offspring were not hampered by traditions and their opportunities were boundless." He portrayed his generation as follows: "They went forth with sound bodies, strength developed in the working of the soil; and if they desired to escape from the drudgery of physical labor, theirs was the world to conquer if they possessed average intelligence, ambition, and industry."[8] Except for the comment about average intelligence, this was a perfect description of Martin and his attitude toward his life.

Franklin described his Grandfather William Martin as "a hard-working farmer, possessed of thrift and good common sense, and

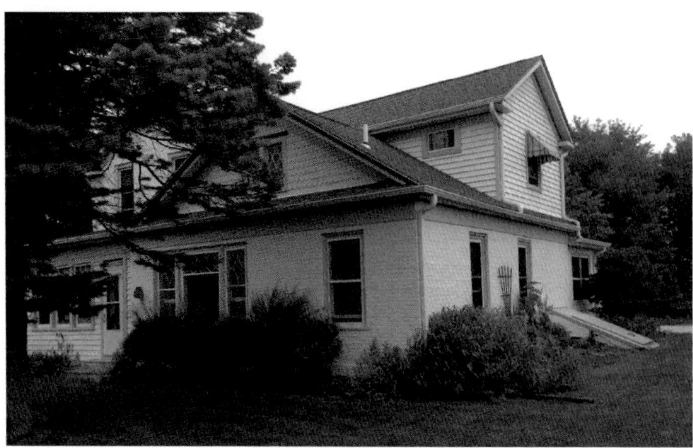

1.10. Recent photo of Franklin's Uncle William Fulmer's home in what is now Lac La Belle, WI.

without too much sentiment" and his Grandmother Caroline Martin as "a slight, vivacious woman, full of strong religious sentiment, and her old family Bible was her only literature." He called hers "a mind with story-telling proclivities, and her histrionic talents were known far and wide." Franklin described his Grandfather Alexander Carlin in great detail. Grandfather Carlin read the current literature and was very opinionated, having an argumentative disposition. Martin said of him, "He was an ardent partisan politician...had adventure, romance, and irrepressible fun in his soul." Martin called his Grandmother Ella Carlin "the steadying influence, the balancing wheel and the financial stabilizer of the Carlin family."[8] It is obvious from these descriptions and other commentaries the tremendous influence his family had on Franklin's character and leadership abilities.

Many members of the Martin family lived on local farms. Lucretia Martin and William Fulmer, and Betsy Martin and William's brother George Fulmer, lived on farms on the banks of Lac La Belle a short distance from the Martin and Carlin homesteads. Permelia Martin had married Luther Hatch and their farm was a mile north of the Martin and Carlin homesteads. Because of the proximity of other Martin family members, there were frequent family gatherings during which the numerous cousins had opportunities to play together in the wonderful surroundings.[9]

In 1862, when Franklin was five years old, his father left to join the Union Army in the Civil War. Franklin and his sister Jeanette (Nettie)

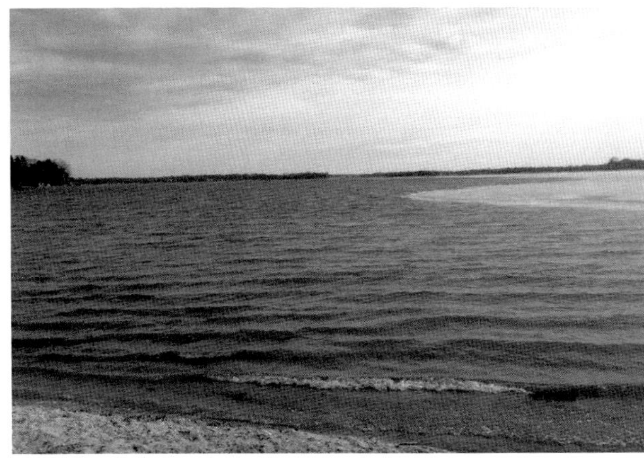

1.11a. Recent photograph of Lac La Belle looking toward Oconomowoc from the area where the Fulmer brickyard was located (details in Chapter 3).

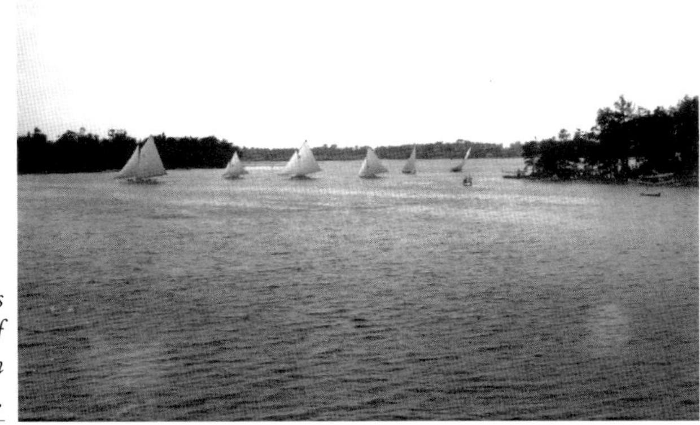

1.11b. Martin's 1918 photograph of Lac La Belle from the brickyard.

(Figure 1.9) and their mother lived in the small home built by his father, surrounded by a large, fertile garden. Extended family and friends cared for the small family. This environment afforded many opportunities for a child to engage in outdoor activities, such as picking berries, nuts, and fruits; fishing in the Rock River; and exploring the surrounding countryside. There were visits to the Fulmer farms (Figure 1.10) on the banks of Lac La Belle, with many cousins as playmates. Spearfishing on Lac La Belle (Figure 1.11) was an especially memorable experience, as was the opportunity to participate in farm work. During these visits, Franklin's musically talented uncles and cousins brought out their instruments and played for everyone's enjoyment.[10]

At the age of five, Franklin worked for his Grandfather Carlin for three cents a day. He traveled on a well-worn mile-and-a-half-long foot-

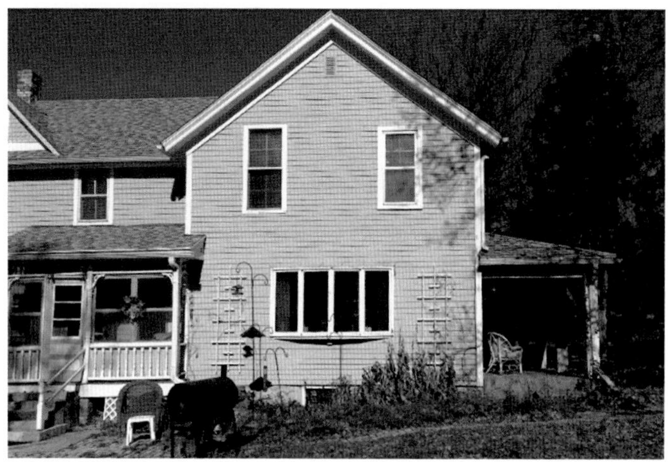

1.12. Recent photograph of Luther and Permelia (Martin) Hatch's home. The criteria used to judge the likelihood that this was the Hatch family home are the same used to evaluate the Carlin home in Figure 1.5.

path twice a day between his home and his grandfather's farm, where his job was to pick up the potatoes his grandfather had dug from the ground. He did this until all the potatoes were harvested. He was quite proud to show his wages to his mother at the end of each day. He took work seriously, a trait that continued during his many years in Wisconsin as a farmhand and laborer. His grandfather said that even at this young age Martin showed a sense of responsibility and worked faithfully at his job every day.[11] This was high praise for a five-year-old boy and a trait that was evident in the physician leader and administrator decades later.

The home of Luther and Permelia Hatch (Figure 1.12) was also a Sunday gathering place for the family. Franklin loved visiting the Hatch farm and playing with his cousins, Alfred and Charles Hatch, in the rolling hills and creeks north of the farm (Figure 1.13).[12]

Father Dies in Civil War

One evening while returning to their home in Ixonia after visiting family in Watertown, the Martins stopped at the township post office in Ixonia to pick up their mail. A letter from a companion of Franklin's

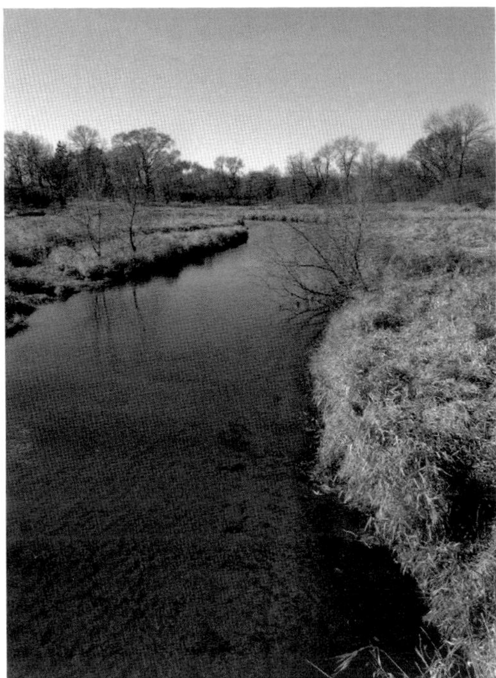

1.13. Recent photograph of the countryside north of the Luther Hatch home, where Franklin and his cousins played and swam during family gatherings.

father informed them of Edmond's death on October 31, 1862, while transferring to a new military camp near Cassville, MO. As happened with many young men who fought in the Civil War, Edmond died of disease rather than battle injuries. Franklin's mother and grandfather wept uncontrollably. On return to Ixonia, the "usually silent" Martin family openly expressed their sympathy and grief. Edmond Martin had been the family favorite and the person that the family believed had a most promising future.[13]

Shortly after his father died, with the help of family and neighbors, the Martin family's small home was enlarged and made more comfortable. Franklin, his sister, and his mother frequently spent time with relatives, including the George Fulmers, the Washington Fulmers, the Luther Hatches, the Richard and Phineas Martins, and the Elon Mungers. These were delightful times for Franklin. Being impatient,

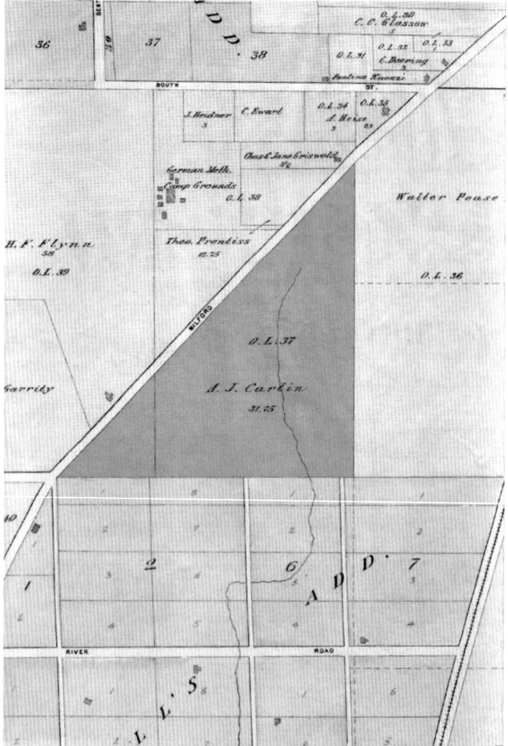

1.14. 1899 plat map of the area of Jefferson County, where Grandfather Carlin's Watertown farm was located.

whenever allowed he ran, never walked, unaccompanied to relatives' farms to play with his cousins. He later said that he continued this practice of rapidly moving from place to place well into his adulthood.[14]

In the winter of 1862–1863, the family went to Watertown, WI, eight miles west of Ixonia, to live with Franklin's maternal aunt, Avaline Carlin Guilder; her husband, Adolphus; and their daughter, Ella. Adolphus became a mentor, and Ella, who was only two years older than Franklin, became a longtime friend. Franklin had daily chores that he took seriously. He made daily trips to pick up milk and the mail. Ella became his constant companion and did her best to guide his daily routine.

Franklin had a memorable Christmas that year at the Guilders' home. He received a dollar bill as a gift from a family friend. At that time, he was interested in drawing and went about creating multiple copies of the dollar that were described by his adult relatives as very good copies. His Uncle Adolphus, however, informed him that what he was doing was creating counterfeit money, a felony. Franklin stopped this endeavor.[15]

Dispute Between Carlins and Martins

In 1864, Franklin's maternal grandparents, Alexander and Ella Carlin, sold their property in Ixonia and moved to a dairy farm in Watertown. This move occurred in part because of a dispute with the Martins over the ownership of a parcel of land on the lot line between their two properties that was covered with valuable hardwood trees. Because of the location, Alexander Carlin had always believed that the land was part of his original tract, but he did not have a survey to prove it. A new survey showed the trees to be on Martin land. According to Franklin Martin, a lack of diplomacy and stubbornness on Grandfather Carlin's part ruined any chance of compromise between the families. The breach was too wide to heal. Interestingly, Grandfather Martin had died in 1861 and the dispute was basically between Grandfather Carlin and the extended Martin family. Perhaps of greater interest, Martin did not mention in his autobiography the untimely death of his Grandfather Martin nor did he mention later in the book the deaths of any of the members of his Wisconsin family. At this juncture the extended Martin family remained in the Ixonia area, while the Carlin family settled in the Watertown area (Figure 1.14). Despite this breach, Franklin and his mother and sister spent many happy times at both the Carlin family farm in Watertown and the homes of the extended Martin family in the Ixonia area.[16]

References

1. Martin, F. H. (1933). *The Joy of Living: An Autobiography,* vol. 1 (pp. 3-4). New York, NY: Doubleday, Doran & Co.
2. Ibid., pp. 4-11.
3. Ibid., pp. 11-13.
4. Ibid., pp. 13-16.
5. Ibid., p. 7.

6. Ibid., pp. 16-18.
7. Ibid., p. 1.
8. Ibid., pp. 18-21.
9. Ibid., pp. 25-27.
10. Ibid., pp. 24-25.
11. Ibid., pp. 27-28.
12. Ibid., pp. 28-29.
13. Ibid., pp. 29-30.
14. Ibid., p. 30.
15. Ibid., pp. 31-33.
16. Ibid., p. 33.

Chapter 2

Childhood: Happy Times

...on moved ov ~~...~~ 8
that the Corliss these thought t
Loustins on Sunday had ... Every ...
claim on the big bend.
the raising on Saturday. Volunteer
~~hands~~ were busy from all the neig...
the week, felling trees, hewing and adjusting ~~the~~ ... Early
...to shape for the new house.
...g of Saturday a dozen or more ...
and boys were on hand to construc...
...ouse. A cellar had been dug in ...
~~...~~ ready to be encased with stone
...alrm logs had been sunk in ...
...ached a bed of solid clay beneath the
...il, lumber had been brought from
...aw mill and a fine lot of dry ...
been contributed by generous neighbors
... ~~...~~ ready to complete with ...
that had been brou...
sturdy oxen
neighbors.

From Boston by common con...
of the guns
...oman for the day. No time was
all directions came the great logs
iron chains about their necks a...
...by of the faithful oxen ... sheep...

HOME LIFE

Although his family was living on a meager income that came mostly from the small government pension his mother received after his father died in the Civil War, Franklin described his childhood as a happy one. His mother's careful financial management meant that their lack of funds did not have a big impact on Franklin or his sister. Relatives, friends, and neighbors helped with his mother's ample, fertile garden and with other tasks.

In Martin's words,

> ...it is my clear recollection that many relatives and neighbors, with their stalwart men, were careful to see that Ed's widow did not want for assistance in the care of her garden, in gathering up her wood, and making such repairs on her little house as required heavy manual labor.[1]

Franklin spent most of his free time outdoors. He said he grew up foraging and ate anything raw or ripe, "including dirt." He reflected:

> If this foraging brought us into touch with ripe or green fruit, of ripe or green nuts, or raw vegetables, we helped ourselves; and not infrequently we paid the penalty of indigestion and severe stomach-aches and cramps that required home remedies and parental sympathy.... It was one of the traditions of our child life...that we must eat a certain amount of common black soil in order to remain healthy. Dirt-eating contests, therefore, were among our daily sport.[1]

Later in life he maintained that it was because he foraged for food and even ate dirt that he had an "immunity" that his pampered colleagues did not have, and that therefore he was less susceptible to "indigestion."

Children in his extended family were expected to behave. They were encouraged to be truthful, obey their elders, not use profanity, not hurt anyone, be peaceful, not steal, and not display unseemly behavior. Punishment for annoying their elders was the switch or flat of the hand.

Franklin recalled that although many of the members of his extended family did not regularly attend church, their values were staunchly Christian and that those mores guided their actions and how they treated others. Only his Grandmother Martin attended church regularly and openly discussed religion with the children. She taught them that the penalty for sinning was an everlasting hell and that the reward for good behavior was the glories of heaven. There was no middle ground in Grandmother Martin's interpretation:

> ...there was but one ultimate penalty for the sinner—a material Hell portrayed with all of the everlasting cruelties, including fire and brimstone, in a vividness of detail that would have made Dante envious. There was but one final reward for those of us who were good—a Heaven, the glories of which contained all of the beauties of Revelation....[1]

These teachings had a profound effect on the young Franklin. When he deceived his mother by skipping Sunday school and instead going to a local strawberry patch with his cousin Alfred Hatch, his mother, quite upset by his deception, punished him with a whipping. On many occasions throughout his life, he was haunted by this experience, and for years he believed that he was doomed to eternal damnation because of this transgression.[1]

Working for Grandfather Carlin

During the summer of 1866, when he was nine years old, Franklin worked on his Grandfather Carlin's farm in Watertown, WI. He guided a horse-drawn corn cultivator and bundled wheat, among numerous other tasks. Guiding a cultivator involved keeping the horse on the right track to avoid trampling the corn. This task was more difficult to accomplish at the end of the rows, where the horse had to be turned about. According to Grandfather Carlin, if plants were trampled it was either Franklin's or the horse's fault, never Grandfather Carlin's. Many

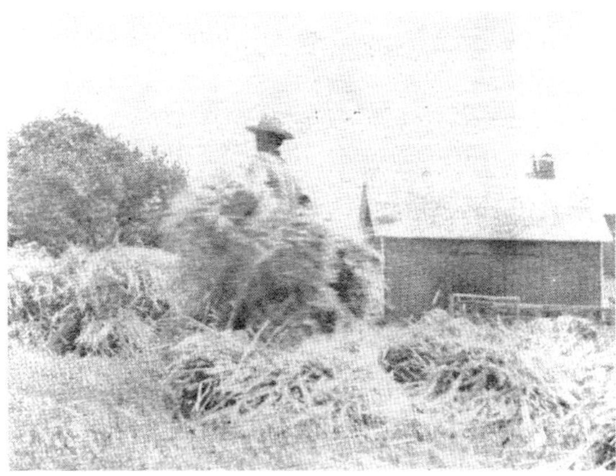

2.1. Man bundling wheat in the 1800s.

farm chores were hard, hot, exhausting work, but Franklin felt that bundling wheat was the worst job, resulting in multiple cuts to the face, hands, and arms (Figure 2.1). Other surgeons, when describing what it was like to be a farm laborer when farming was done manually, agree with Martin's assessment that bundling and shocking wheat was the worst job on a farm.[2]

Harvesting wheat was a multi-step process. First, his grandfather and one of the hired hands cut the wheat with a cradle scythe using long, sweeping cuts close to the ground. Then two other hired hands gathered the wheat into sheaves with hand rakes and secured it into bundles. The bundles were then gathered into groups of 12. Ten of the bundles were stood on end and pressed together into the shocks. The shocks were then capped by two bundles of wheat to protect the shocks from the rain while they dried for several days.

Gathering the bundles into shocks was Franklin's job. Despite disliking many of the chores he was asked to perform, Franklin wanted to succeed and please his grandfather, so he worked hard to perform to the best of his ability. He reflected later in life that this work he did for his grandfather, unpleasant as it was, taught him to be responsible and hard working even under the harshest of circumstances. Of Grandfather Carlin's attitude about work Martin said, "Grandfather made play of work, and instilled a spirit of contest in all who worked with him."[3] This theme would remain with Martin for the rest of his life and have an impact on his feelings about working with others.

At midday all fieldwork ceased, and Grandmother Carlin and Aunt Mary brought out a hearty meal of sandwiches, milk, donuts, and much more, as was the custom in those times and continues up to the present in many farm families.[3] I recently helped a cousin harvest field corn, and his mother brought lunch out to the field for us almost every day. It gave us a short respite from our labor and the opportunity to return to work quickly and energized. What a wonderful tradition.

As described earlier, in the mid- to late 1800s the harvesting of crops on small farms in the area where Franklin grew up was done entirely by hand. Stationary threshing machines were transported from farm to farm to thresh the wheat and oats: "Nothing quite equalled the excitement of threshing time—mysterious machinery to watch, ...the bubbling good nature and bantering antics of good fellowship."[3] Even in the first half of the 20th century, horse-drawn farm equipment was the best many owners of small farms could afford. I spoke recently with local farmers from the area where Franklin grew up, who pointed out that it was not until after World War II that all-purpose, rubber-tired tractors became readily available to farmers in this area.

During World War II, because manufacturers were almost exclusively producing vehicles for the war, new tractors were unavailable. Many of the farmers I talked with had experience with the harvesting of oats and corn as late as the 1940s without the benefit of balers and threshing machines. They verified what Franklin had said, that harvesting wheat was hot, exhausting work. One farmer added that after spending a day harvesting wheat by hand "you itched everywhere."

It was not until the 1950s that the number of tractors on farms in the U.S. exceeded the number of horses and mules. Farmers who are now in their 90s, who grew up in the 1930s and 1940s in the same area as Franklin Martin, remember well what it was like to farm when everything was either done by hand or with horse-drawn equipment. Even with the advent of tractors, balers, and threshing machines, some harvesting tasks were still done by hand on small farms until the 1950s.

BARGAINING WITH GRANDFATHER CARLIN

At the end of the summer, Franklin bargained with his Grandfather Carlin about his pay. He wanted some cash to purchase clothes to help relieve his mother of the responsibility of clothing him and to purchase

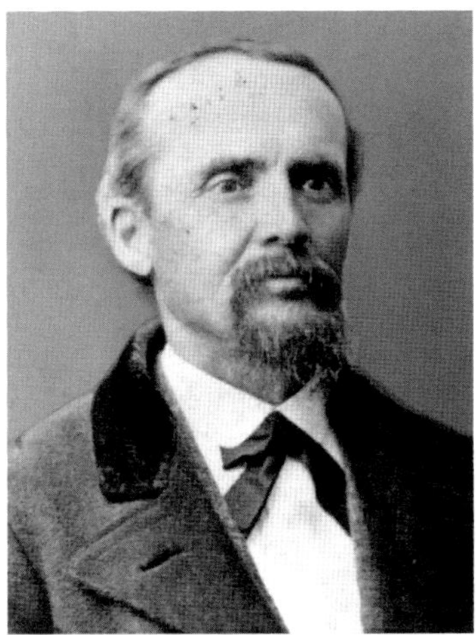

2.2. Elon Munger, Franklin's stepfather.

an ewe from his grandfather, which, along with her offspring, he would keep on his grandfather's farm. After extensive discussions, serious negotiations, and with the encouragement of the sympathetic women of the family, Grandmother Carlin and Aunt Mary, his grandfather eventually accepted the proposition. Two years later, Franklin owned nine sheep. But Grandfather Carlin believed nine-year-old Franklin had taken advantage of him; he was somewhat embarrassed that the transactions had resulted in Franklin owning one-fourth of the sheep on the farm. Under pressure, Franklin sold all but one sheep. Looking back on these times in his autobiography, Martin credited this experience with helping him to learn to transact financial deals, industriously busy himself, and make every working task a game.[4]

Franklin's Mother Marries Uncle Elon Munger

In 1867, after a short courtship, Franklin's mother remarried—some five years after Franklin's father died in the war. She married Franklin's Uncle Elon Munger (Figure 2.2), whose first wife, Terressa Martin—Franklin's father's sister—had died. Elon had four children ranging in age from six to 13 years old, all of whom had been adopted by families who wanted to keep them. Elon was a master carpenter, an avid reader, and a good father. The family moved to Milwaukee, where Elon had

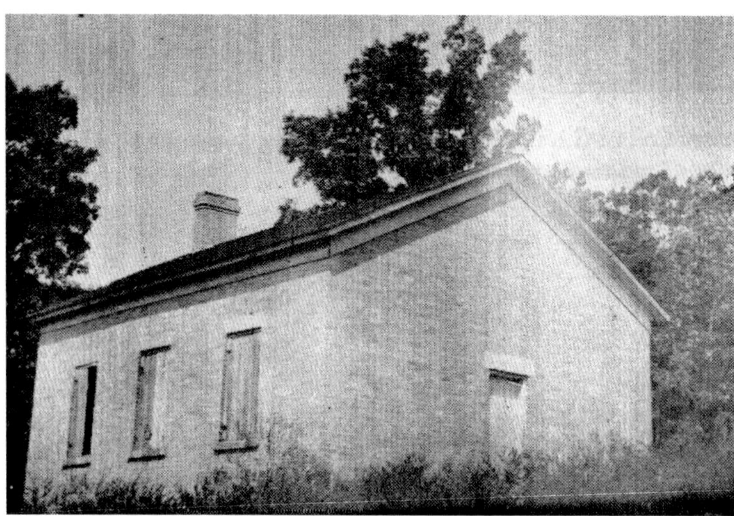

2.3. Woodlawn School in Ixonia, WI, on the corner of Ski Slide and Lang Roads, where Franklin attended school until age 10.

found better employment. They lived there for two years, during which time Franklin attended Milwaukee schools.[5]

In the spring of 1869, the family moved to the growing village of Oconomowoc, near Ixonia, where Elon found new employment. Elon purchased a tract of land at the edge of town and in time built a small home. These were prosperous times for the family and a chance for young Franklin to learn new skills. Elon taught Franklin carpentry and masonry, which served him well in the following years. During summers at this stage of his life, Franklin again worked on the Carlin farm, but also on the farms of his uncles, William and George Fulmer.[6]

It was at this time that Franklin's half-sister Jenny Ada Munger was born, followed three years later by the birth of a half-brother, Carlin Munger. Franklin described his family life during these times as "imbued by wholesome living, daily tasks, and unostentatious belief in common honesty and filial love."[7]

One day while Franklin was weeding the family garden, a neighbor noticed his abilities and offered him a job weeding and caring for her garden. The news of his work ethic spread to other neighbors, who requested he work in their gardens. He also performed other jobs, including chopping wood, to earn spending money. In addition, he became head janitor at his school. It was already apparent by the age

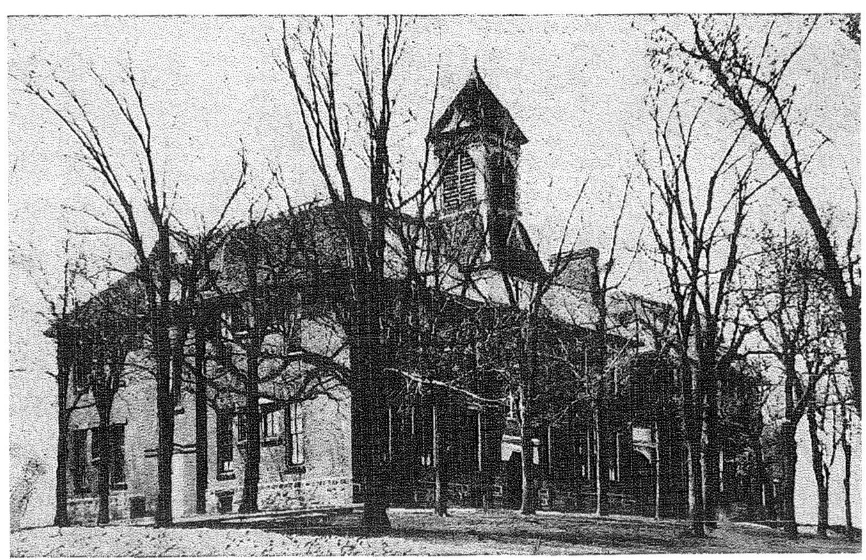

2.4. Elroy Seminary, Elroy, WI.

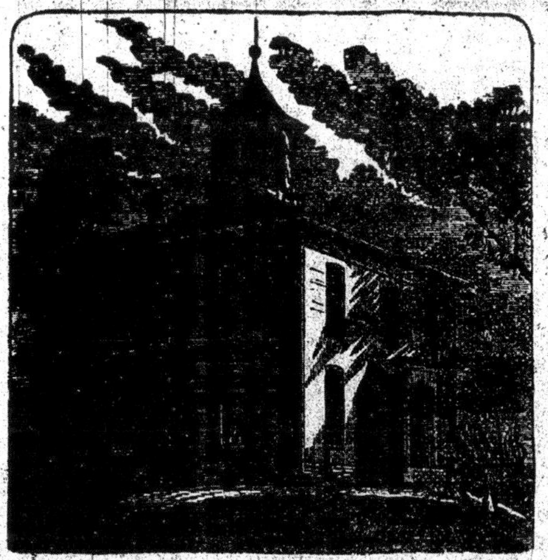

Elroy Seminary, Elroy, Juneau Co., Wis.

A christian institution of learning for the education of both sexes, having the same courses of study, Classical and Scientific, for both ladies and gentlemen.

It is believed that this institution ranks among the best Academies of the country, and efforts are being made continually to increase its facilities.

A thoroughly organized commercial department is also connected with the school.

Fall Term begins August 26.

FACULTY.

Rev. F. M. Washburn, A. B. Principal.

C. E. Booth, M. D. Professor of Anatomy and Physiology.

Martha A. Washburn, M. A., Lady Principal.

Anna M. Hopper, Teacher of German and Mathematics.

Eva Brown, Principal Primary Department.

Victoria P. Bovee, Principal Commercial Department.

Genie McClure, Teacher of Music.

of 12 that Franklin was always capable of finding jobs to occupy his time and give him spending money.[8] In the words of one family member, "...Franklin developed into a ruddy, sturdy, industrious lad, receiving his elementary education by the sweat of his brow."[9]

Education from Ages Four through 16

From ages four to 10 Franklin was a student at a district school in Ixonia (Figure 2.3). He said that he was not a serious student during this time and was known for his mischief in class. In Martin's words, "The only pleasure of my early school days was in the play hours, and in mischief-making during the long sessions of instruction."[10] His best descriptions of his youth are the ones about his outdoor games and adventures both with his school friends and on his own.

From age 11 to 15 he attended classes in Milwaukee, Oconomowoc, and Minneapolis schools and believed that this is when he was slowly becoming a "serious" student. At age 11, in Franklin's second year (1868–1869) as a student in a Milwaukee primary school, his behavior in the classroom began to change significantly. His new teacher stressed that she was dependent on her students' reliability. With this covenant, Franklin became a model student for the first time and in his words, "...that winter of schooling stands out in my primary school life as the one most satisfactory in the point of knowledge gained. School was revealed...as something serious and worth while."[5]

In his next two years of schooling in Oconomowoc, he had an equally impactful teacher, Mr. D. B. Smith, who, along with teaching the usual subjects, gave personal talks about conduct, the fundamentals of daily living, and other practical subjects. These subjects made for improved discipline and character in his students. Also, "...he introduced a number of competitive tasks that sharpened our intellects and interested us in our work."[11]

In 1873, at age 16, Franklin entered the Elroy Seminary (Figure 2.4) in Elroy, WI, 100 miles northwest of the Ixonia/Oconomowoc area. His family had moved to the area because of better employment opportunities for Elon. The school had an academic atmosphere and a spirit of earnestness that encouraged ambitious and serious study. The curriculum included social and religious training in addition to the standard courses. Franklin was drawn to a course in physiology taught by Dr. Charles Booth, a

2.5. Pages from Franklin's Elroy Seminary notebook with his notes on digestion, circulation, the heart, and the nervous system.

local physician. As demonstrated in one of Franklin's notebooks from his studies at the seminary, he had a keen interest in this course (Figure 2.5). From all appearances Franklin's studies at the Elroy Seminary had a significant impact on his intellectual development, as demonstrated by two compositions in his Elroy Seminary notebook. The first, "Keep Balanced," reads as follows (original spelling and punctuation retained):

> To keep Balanced is easy enough if you know how.
> In the first place to keep your brain balanced you must
> sleep as many hours in the day as you work or play.
> To keep your body balanced you must wear big boots.
> To keep your head balanced you must join the good templars.
> Do not let your tongue out balance your brain.
> Do not let your clothes out balance your pocketbook.
> Do not spend your money before you earn it, or what
> you spend may out balance what you earn.
> I must stop or I fear my foolishness will out balance your patients.
> —Written by F. H. Martin Dec. 10th .74[12]

Although a less-than-erudite composition, it still demonstrates an early attempt on his part to put some scholarly thoughts into words. When one realizes that his education up to this point was unexceptional, this composition demonstrates a great leap forward.

The next untitled composition in his notebook is even more impressive. It is a poem he wrote about an early Civil War battle, the battle of Wilson's Creek, that occurred August 10, 1861, near Springfield, MO. Martin's father died a year later at a military camp in Cassville, MO, a few miles from the battlefield. Almost certainly his interest in the battle of Wilson's Creek was related to his father's untimely death nearby. Martin must have studied the battle in detail because his description of what occurred that fateful day is basically correct (original spelling and punctuation retained):[13]

> It was August tenth eighteen-sixty one,
> But just the day before, they had made the enemy run.
>
> This day the leaden rain was falling,
> And the canon bawls were brawling.

That day many a brave soul fled,
But they went to a glorious land over head,

Among the souls that fled that day,
Is one that we will remember, as long as we stay.

This day that face looked very sad,
Nevertheless they fought like mad.

We did not no, where the enemy had got
The General rideing forward, his horse was shot.

There he stood with his hand upon his head
Looking about upon the wounded and the dead.

One of his staff asked him if he was hurt,
He said—"not so much but that I can work,"

He mounted another horse, and rode through the storm again
Through the ranks and shot and shell and leaden rain and stain.

At the time the battle was raging large
The men were preparing to make a charge

They said who will go a-head to take the lead,
We'll have, General Lyon with his brilliant steed.

So he went forward with that desperate charge,
And it was the last time he led his men at large.

With one eye upon the rebels, and the other on the rest,
Alas! a ball entered that brave old breast.

He was caught in the arms of those that loved him dear,
And was carried from the field with many a tear.

His brave body was carried home with military order,
But not without tears and some disorder.

His soul left him just about dark,
But now he is traveling in a heavenly park.

People? Nation? Remember that day,
Old, and young, and even the gray.

—F. H. Martin[14]

Although not necessarily an excellent poem, it demonstrates Franklin's growing intellect and is worthy of examination. One must remember that the year before attending the Elroy Seminary he was working in his uncle's mill in Minneapolis and attending Minneapolis public schools. In the years leading up to attending medical school in Chicago, IL, he was already becoming a thoughtful, intelligent individual.

While attending the Elroy Seminary, Franklin decided he wanted to be a teacher. In 1874, at age 16, he passed the teacher examination for Juneau County and took a teaching position that summer in Mauston, WI, 10 miles from Elroy. At that time, each county had its own examination and issued a teaching certificate that was only good for that county. In addition to his instructor duties, he used the carpentry skills that Elon had taught him to make repairs at the school.

While teaching at the Mauston school he stayed with the Goodman family in an area surrounded by extraordinary and beautiful countryside that was inspiring to him. He said of his experiences there,

> In the hectic days of later life, when the taskmaster was strenuous in his driving, I thought of the wonderful pastoral picture on the Goodman farm, where leisure and beauty were my playmates. Never have there been more wonderful skies, sunshine, or bird life, nor has there ever been greater appreciation.[15]

Regrettably, Franklin found his teaching experience less inspiring. Except for one student, he felt he had little impact on his young charges, who he believed were not motivated to learn. He took great satisfaction from the one boy on whom he felt he had made an impression. In his free time, he expanded his horizons reading about Napoleon and the French Revolution—topics he later returned to during his time in Chicago.[15]

Because his family was unable to provide Franklin with funds for his school expenses, he devised a new scheme for earning money. He arranged for a teamster to haul oak logs from the family's tract of land outside Mauston to Elroy, where he sold them for $1 each. This transaction was yet another example of his entrepreneurial and organizational abilities, which gave him great pride and served him well throughout his life.[16]

References

1. Martin, F. H. (1933). *The Joy of Living: An Autobiography*, vol. 1 (pp. 36-39). New York, NY: Doubleday, Doran & Co.
2. Connaughton, D. (1991). *Warren Cole, MD, and the Ascent of Scientific Surgery* (pp. 15-16). Chicago, IL: The Warren and Clara Cole Foundation.
3. Martin, F. H. (1933). *The Joy of Living: An Autobiography*, vol. 1 (pp. 39-42). New York, NY: Doubleday, Doran & Co.
4. Ibid., pp. 45-47.
5. Ibid., pp. 54-56.
6. Ibid., pp. 57-58.
7. Ibid., p. 59.
8. Ibid., pp. 59-62.
9. Cubbins, W. (1935). Franklin H. Martin. *Bull Am Coll Surg*, 20(2), 39-40.
10. Martin, F. H. (1933). *The Joy of Living: An Autobiography*, vol 1 (pp. 48-49). New York, NY: Doubleday, Doran & Co.
11. Ibid., pp. 65-66.
12. Martin, F. H. (1874). *Unpublished Elroy Seminary notebook*, p. 26. In: Franklin Martin Collection, Archives of the American College of Surgeons, Chicago, IL.
13. Foote, S. (1986). *The Civil War: A Narrative, Vol. I. Fort Sumter to Perryville* (pp. 91-95). New York, NY: Random House, Inc.
14. Martin, F. H. *Unpublished Elroy Seminary notebook*. 1874, pp. 35-37. In: Franklin Martin Collection, Archives of the American College of Surgeons, Chicago, IL.
15. Martin, F. H. (1933). *The Joy of Living: An Autobiography*, vol. 1 (pp. 77-86). New York, NY: Doubleday, Doran & Co.
16. Ibid., pp. 104-105.

Chapter 3

Early Work Experience

oon moved ov... those ~~[struck]~~ thought it

that the Corliss house had brought

visitors on Sunday had. Everybo...

claim on the big land.

the raising on Saturday. Volunteers

~~[struck]~~ were busy from all the neig...

the week, felling trees, and hewing addition... Early

the shape for the new house.

g of Saturday a dozen or more str...

nd boys were on hand to construc...

house. A cellar had been dug in th...

~~[struck]~~ ready to be encased with ston...

atin logs had been sunk in ben...

reached a bed of solid clay beneath the

il, lumber had been brought from

ow mill and a fine lot of dry o...

been contributed by generous neighbors

en ~~[struck]~~ ready to compete with Se...

sturdy oxen that had been brou...

neighbors.

Then Morton by common cons...

...oeman of the guns for the day. No time was

all directions came the great logs

...on chains about their necks a...

... of the faithful oxen

... of ... sheep...

Uncle Adolphus Guilder's Mill

Adolphus Guilder, Franklin's maternal uncle (Figure 3.1), had perfected a process for purifying flour. In 1872, when Franklin was 14 years old, his uncle invited Franklin to become an apprentice in his Minneapolis, MN, plant. Franklin was hesitant to accept. He had no big-city experience, and it pained him to meet strangers. He said, "I was tongue-tied in their presence. I could work, I was most ambitious, I enjoyed my own people, and above all I loved fun and frolics; but I was paralyzed with bashfulness until an acquaintanceship was somewhat prolonged."[1] He thought himself a poor conversationalist and had developed an appearance of bravado, brusqueness, and abruptness to compensate for his social unease. Martin believed his response to strangers distressed his family and friends, and this embarrassed him. Nevertheless, he accepted the offer and went to live with the Guilders.

Adolphus's wife, Avaline Carlin Guilder, had died and Franklin's maternal aunt, Mary Carlin, whom everyone in the family loved, had come to Minneapolis to live with the Guilders and to be the chaperone and companion of her niece Ella, a pleasant young lady who was entering society. Aunt Mary and Cousin Ella, whom Franklin was convinced had orchestrated the plan to have him come to Minneapolis, took on the task of "civilizing" Franklin and breaking down his reserve. Franklin felt that, "At times they must have been discouraged to the point of abandoning the task; but I showed in my shy way my love for them."[1] Ella's friends also helped Franklin to improve his response to strangers. By his own analysis, Franklin was painfully shy and introverted. He worked his entire life at overcoming his difficulty interacting with strangers. His discomfort lessened but never disappeared completely.[1]

Uncle Adolphus was an inventor and in Franklin's estimation a genius. He was interested in the process of milling wheat into flour. He had perfected the middlings purifier, which made it feasible to separate the wheat bran from the wheat flour without losing large amounts of

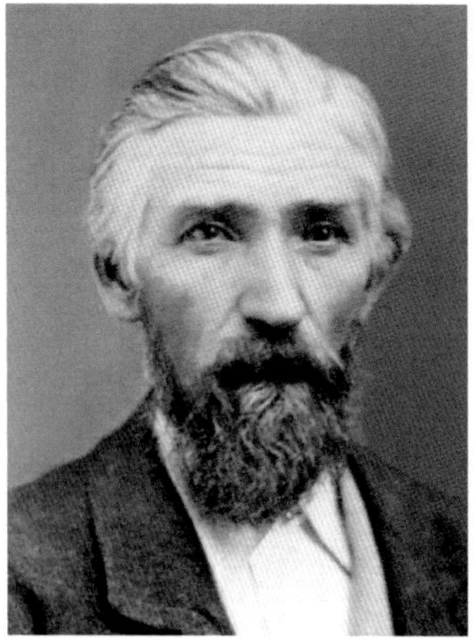

3.1. Uncle Adolphus Guilder, Franklin's mentor when he worked in the flour mill.

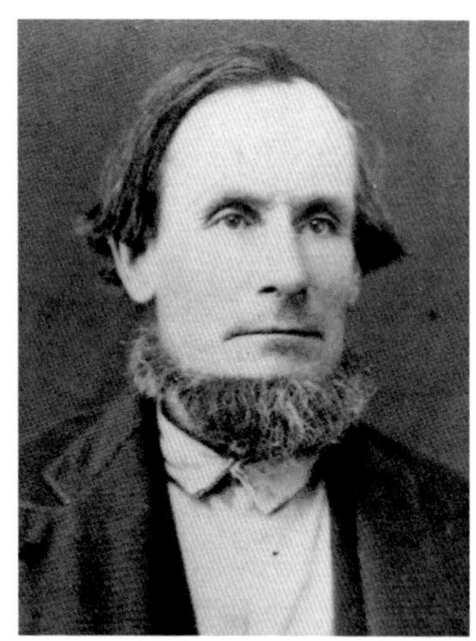

3.2. Uncle George Fulmer, owner of the Fulmer brickyard.

flour. This capability was achieved by use of a graduated set of sieves that made it possible to separate the middlings—the coarser particles of the ground wheat—leaving a finer grade of flour. The finest grade of flour that remained after passing through the last sieve was almost pure white flour. This process made commercial milling more profitable because it produced larger quantities of high-grade white flour. Another innovation, the steel wheat grinder, also had recently been introduced. Steel wheat grinders replaced the more cumbersome stone grinders.

Adolphus's plant manufactured the new middlings flour purifier and milled flour. After other mills, like Pillsbury, failed in their attempts to purchase the patent from Mr. Guilder, they sought to imitate his process, but he prevailed in court. Consequently, the perfected middlings purifier was in great demand. Minneapolis was in the wheat belt and was becoming a flour milling center, raising demand further. At the time Franklin began his apprenticeship, the Guilder plant was extremely busy producing the middlings purifier, enlarging the factory's capacity, and remodeling other mills in preparation for installing the new purifiers.

On his arrival at the plant, Franklin was appointed as a handyman, and in that position he mastered the principles and mechanics of all the machines. This approach was typical of how Franklin undertook any new task. Knowing how machinery worked and the reason for each step in a process was essential to him. In my experience, this intellectual curiosity is quite typical of individuals raised in a rural environment, especially in the late 19th and early 20th centuries. To succeed in their livelihood, they needed to understand the workings and repair of their machinery in detail, as hiring a mechanic to fix broken equipment would be both time-consuming and expensive. Frequently it took a mechanic many weeks to repair a piece of equipment because of delays awaiting the arrival of new parts.

One of Franklin's early assignments at the plant was to be the handyman for a group that was installing new middlings purifiers in Pillsbury Company mills in Minneapolis and other sites. Soon thereafter, at the age of 15, Franklin became a supervisor and oversaw the installation of milling machines. An example of his industriousness is his response when he discovered that the "stone pickers," the men who overhauled and redressed the stones used to grind the wheat, needed better pick handles. The process of redressing the stones was necessary when the stones were no longer able to effectively grind the wheat into flour, and it was essential that the picks be kept in good condition. The steel pick had to be kept sharp and the wood handles had to be carefully chosen.[2]

From his observation of the stone pickers at work, Franklin appreciated that they preferred white hickory for the handles—the same wood Franklin's family in Wisconsin used for axe handles. After an exchange of letters with his cousins in Ixonia, Franklin started a successful business providing the stone pickers with white hickory handles. His cousins in Ixonia cut the white hickory to the appropriate size, and Franklin turned the wood into handles on a lathe at his uncle's plant.

The Guilder plant and its new milling process were becoming well known in Europe and, much to Adolphus Guilder's delight, European mill owners began visiting the Minneapolis plant. He thoroughly enjoyed demonstrating and describing how his new purifier worked.[3]

After a summer of hard work in the mill, Franklin enrolled in a Minneapolis public school. The following spring, he became ill with typhoid fever but recovered and returned to mill work. Re-exposure to the mill dust exacerbated his bronchial cough and fevers, and respiratory problems necessitated his return to Wisconsin. His physical condition prohibited him from working that summer, but by fall he had returned to his usual good health and was able to attend school at the Elroy Seminary in Wisconsin.[4]

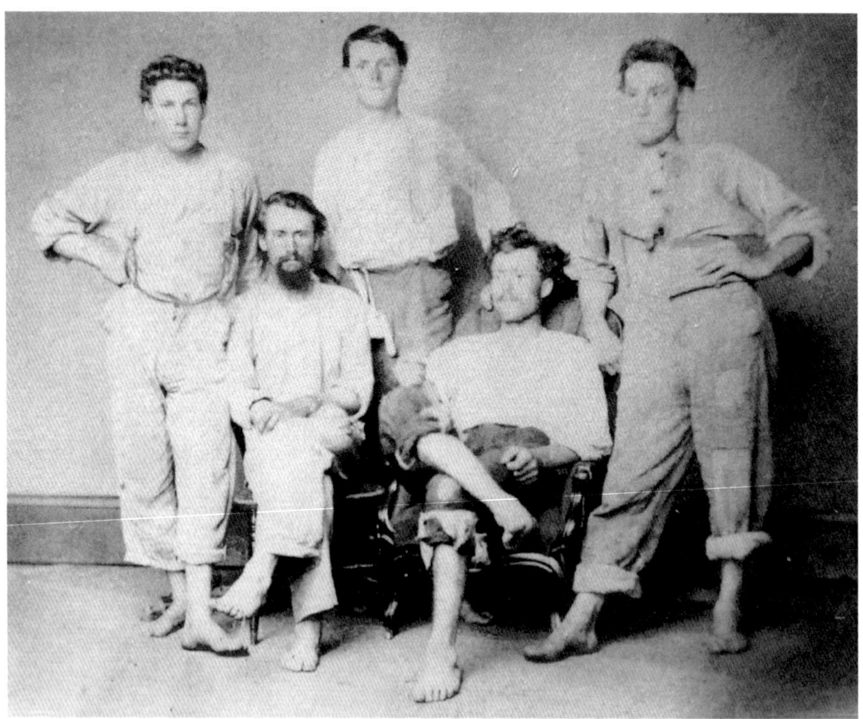

3.3. Fulmer brickyard crew. From left: Franklin Martin, Julius Besendorf, Thomas Fulmer, Richard Fulmer, and Washington Fulmer. The three Fulmers were Franklin's cousins.

Summer Work at the Fulmer Brickyard

After completing his schooling for the year at the Elroy Seminary and teaching a term at the Mauston Public School, Franklin needed employment for the summer of 1875. He wrote his Uncle George Fulmer (Figure 3.2), who owned a successful brickyard on Lac La Belle opposite the town of Oconomowoc and requested that he be considered for employment as a worker in the brickyard. His uncle replied that he would hire Franklin if he believed he was strong enough to handle the strenuous work. Based on his experience, Franklin believed he would be able to perform the required physical labor and replied that he would report for work in early July. He would be working with his cousins Thomas, Richard, and Washington Fulmer, along with Julius Besendorf, the hired helper (Figure 3.3).

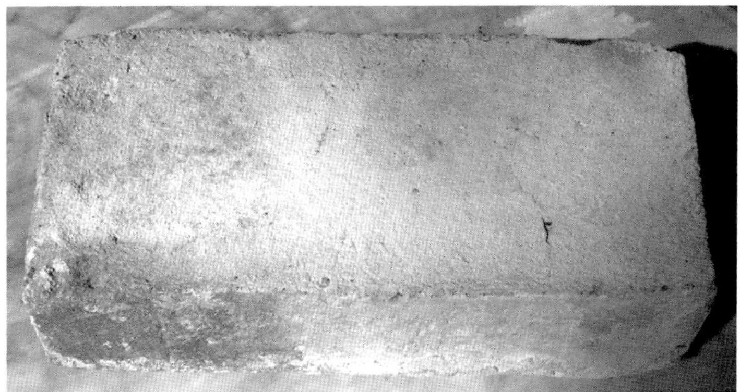

3.4. Brick from the Fulmer brickyard. Gift from Tim and Rose Burns, who now own Martin's Uncle William Fulmer's home where the bricks were found. The color and style of the brick are consistent with the type of bricks made in the Fulmer brickyard.

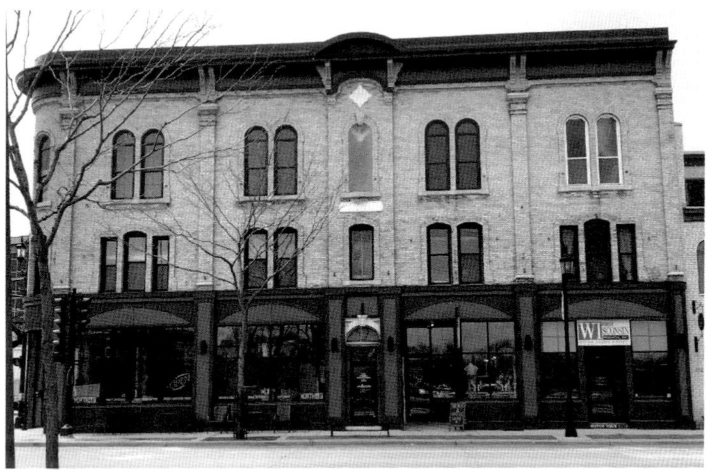

3.5. Flanagan Building in downtown Oconomowoc, WI, which was constructed with Fulmer brick. The building is unusual because of its arched brick window casings. The Fulmer brickyard was the only local brickyard where beveled brick molds were used to make the bricks necessary to construct arched window casings.

Brickmaking was a multi-step process—all of which were strenuous. First, the clay used to make the bricks was dug from a 25-foot-deep pit that was five feet below ground water level at its deepest point. The dripping clay was transported in wheelbarrows along wood plank tracks to the processing yard. The clay was then shoveled into the mixing pit, where a horse pulled a large paddle in circles to mix the clay. The clay mixture was then placed in wooden molds with six slots in each mold. The molds, which weighed 40 pounds when filled with clay, were carried to the drying yard. Once the clay was dry enough, the molds were placed on their sides and left for further drying. Next, they were placed in wooden frames with coverings for the final drying step. After several days of drying, the bricks were removed from the molds. They were transported to the kiln and fired, a process that took two weeks and converted the bricks into the final product. The resulting bricks were 8 x 4 x 2″ in size. With two kilns the brickmakers were able to produce 300,000 bricks each year. After each use the molds were dipped in water and coated on the inside with fine sand to prevent the clay from sticking to the mold. Once the firing process was completed, the bricks were loaded onto wagons and hauled to Oconomowoc for their use in fabricating new buildings. Many of the businesses and homes in Oconomowoc and many other nearby communities were constructed of Fulmer brick that Martin participated in making[5] (Figures. 3.4 and 3.5).

In Franklin's own words, each of the steps involved in brickmaking required "backbreaking labor." Early in his work at the brickyard, he frequently was so exhausted that he could not work at all, and one of his cousins would send him back to the house to recover. He slowly acclimated, however, and became a valued member of the team, later saying, "I suffered many hours of depression and near despair during the first two weeks of this labor, before I attained a physical condition that made it possible for me to enjoy my work, and the assurance that I was a valuable and normal workman."[5]

Ultimately Franklin adapted to the routine and, in the end, found the brickyard an enjoyable place to work. He described brickmaking as a strenuous but delightful job. He said of his work with his cousins, "With our well-fed bodies, and with the joy of an active life and youth in our souls, we were indeed a happy group."[5]

Martin described the impact of the manual labor he performed in his younger years on his later life: "Many times, in my life, when my strength has been tried to the breaking point, I have obtained sustaining power by reminiscing on those first days in the brickyard and the harvest field, when I was fatigued to the limit of endurance and had no reserve force."[5] When one understands the strenuous labor that was required to make bricks and harvest wheat in the 1870s, it is quite apparent that such arduous work significantly affected his character and self-confidence.

Although in the right circumstances Franklin enjoyed strenuous labor, especially when working with his cousins and other young men, he ultimately yearned to avoid spending his entire life doing such work. He said of the time he spent in the fields and the brickyard with his cousins, "...the joyous memory of precious days, of companionship with honest men engaged in physical labor, and of competitive tasks which Nature impelled in the out-of-doors of a choice region of Wisconsin, my birthplace."[6]

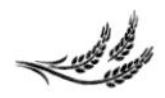

References

1. Martin, F. H. (1933). *The Joy of Living: An Autobiography*, vol. 1 (pp. 67-69). New York, NY: Doubleday, Doran & Co.
2. Ibid., pp. 70-71.
3. Ibid., pp. 71-73.
4. Ibid., pp. 73-77.
5. Ibid., pp. 91-100.
6. Ibid., p. vii.

Chapter 4

"I Will Be a Doctor"

oon moved so those ~~[illegible]~~ thought

that the Corbins had

visitors on Sunday. Every

claim on the big bend.

the raising on Saturday. Volunteers

~~hands~~ were busy from all the neig

the week, felling trees, hewing and adzing ~~the~~

in shape for the new house. Early

g of Saturday a dozen or more

and boys were on hand to construct

house. ~~a~~ A cellar had been dug in

~~[illegible]~~ ready to be encased with stone

logs had been sunk in

reached a bed of solid clay beneath the

il, lumber had been brought from

saw mill and a fine lot of dry

been contributed by generous neighbors

~~oxen~~ ready to compete with

sturdy oxen that had been brou

neighbors.

Joe Mosher by common cons

for the day. No time was

of the yoke

all directions came the great logs

iron chains about their necks

of the faithful oxen

Summer Job Working on the Russell Farm

In 1876 at age 18, Franklin took a summer job harvesting grain, among many other responsibilities, on the Russell farm in Concord, WI, three miles south of Ixonia. Arthur Russell, an old friend of the Martin family and a respected member of the community, offered Franklin a job as a farmhand based on his reputation as an excellent worker. He was to receive $2 a day plus board and lodging. The Russell farm, with its large home and up-to-date barns and equipment, was an enjoyable place to work. Russell's attractive 18-year-old daughter and a school friend were spending the summer on the farm and Franklin fully enjoyed the opportunities he had to unwind with them after a hard day's labor.

As described earlier, harvesting grain in the 1800s in late summer was hot, exhausting work. First, the oats were cut and gathered into bundles. The stiff, cut ends of the oats cut the face, hands, and arms. On a particularly hot day in early August, while binding the oats, an event occurred that changed Franklin's life. He had stopped at the end of a row to rest (Figure 4.1). From there he saw a man dressed in white linen riding leisurely in a horse-drawn buggy along the shaded road. That man was Dr. Daniel McLaren Miller, Oconomowoc's most respected family physician. His buggy had a white canvas top with open sides, and the horse was protected by a white fly net. Franklin said he felt joy and envy. He gazed at Dr. Miller riding by and thought, "Yes, I will be a doctor. Why haven't I thought of it before?"[1]

Making Plans to Become a Doctor

Anxious to put his plan into action, after dinner that evening Franklin all but ran the three miles to the Oconomowoc post office, where he purchased stationery and wrote to his Aunt Mary Carlin (Figure 4.2) in Watertown of his plans to become a doctor. He wanted to move to Watertown, live in his grandfather's house for the winter, and be proc-

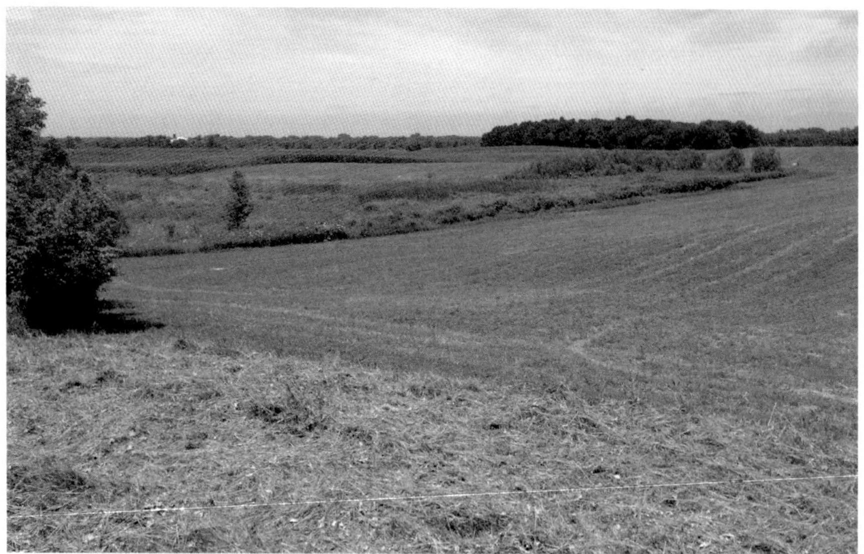

4.1. Field where Franklin was binding oats when he saw Dr. Daniel McLaren Miller drive by in his buggy.

tored by Dr. William Spalding, a prominent Watertown physician. He requested that Aunt Mary make the arrangements. He wanted to be free of the drudgery of manual labor. In a matter of hours, Franklin had developed and implemented a plan that most people would have spent weeks creating. In two days, Aunt Mary's return letter informed him that Dr. Spalding had agreed to his proposal but wanted to speak with Franklin before making formal arrangements. Dr. Spalding requested that in exchange for proctoring, Franklin would tend the office fires and clean the office.

Aunt Mary was both proud and anxious about his new plans. She was concerned about the cost of medical school, the many years of study, the hard life and long hours of a physician, the possibility of exposure to dreaded diseases, and much more. He was unperturbed by her concerns and believed that this career was his destiny. Later he talked to his mother and sister Nettie, who approved of his plans. His stepfather Elon did not display enthusiasm for the venture, but he did not discourage him.[2]

Once the Russell harvest was completed, Franklin returned to work at the Fulmer brickyard with his cousins, where he spent the remain-

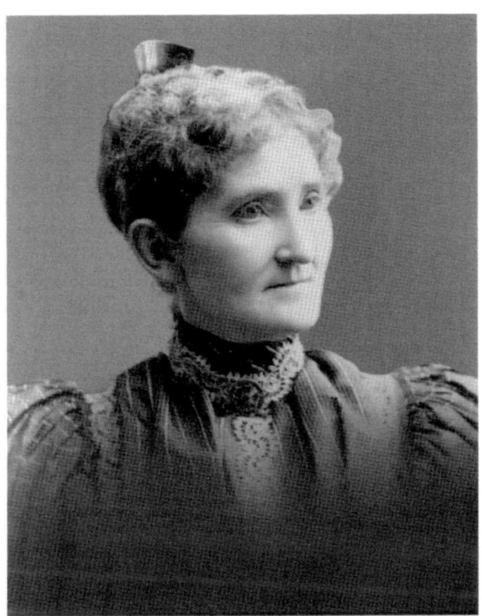

4.2. Aunt Mary Carlin, Martin's supportive maternal aunt.

der of the summer of 1876 earning additional funds for medical school expenses. He continued to enjoy working and socializing with his cousins and with his Aunt Betsy and Uncle George Fulmer and their daughters. He realized he would miss working in the open air and the wonderful surroundings on the shores of Lac La Belle, with its brilliant sunrises and sunsets. He stated that he left there in perfect health, with a well-tuned body. But at the end of October it was time for him to move to the Carlin farm in Watertown and begin his preceptorship with Dr. Spalding.[3]

By prior agreement, in exchange for his room and board at Grandfather Carlin's farm, he was to perform daily chores. He was to keep wood on hand in the kitchen, dining room, and living room. The fires in those rooms were to be started at 5:00 am. Daily, the horses were to be watered and fed, their stables kept clean, and their coats brushed. The cows had to be milked, put in their stalls, fed nightly, and put out every morning. The beef cattle and the hogs also had to be fed and watered daily. As was his habit, Franklin designed a routine for completing his daily tasks efficiently so he could join the family for breakfast before heading to Dr. Spalding's office.[4]

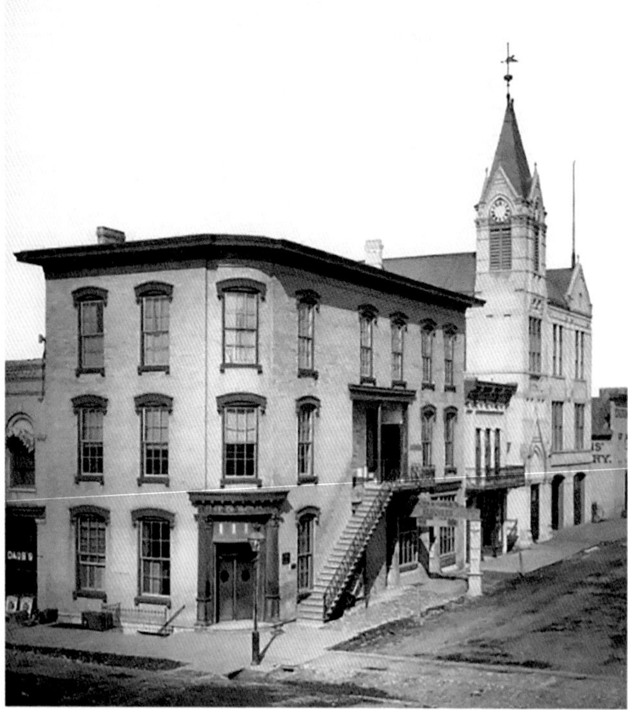

4.3. Watertown Bank Building in the late 1800s. Dr. William Spalding's office, where Franklin apprenticed, was on the second floor.

PRECEPTORSHIP WITH DR. SPALDING

Franklin was scheduled to meet Dr. Spalding for the first time on a Monday morning at the physician's second-floor office in the Watertown Bank Building (Figure 4.3). When Franklin arrived, there was no fire, so he built one and warmed up the office. On arrival, Dr. Spalding questioned Franklin's desire to become a doctor. Spalding seemed disappointed with Franklin's youth and apparent inexperience. They agreed that Franklin would study from 9:00 am to 3:00 pm and that he would keep the fires and sweep the floors. Although Franklin thought that the office would benefit from a good cleaning, Dr. Spalding did not want things disturbed.

Spalding went to his bookcase and brought out *Wilson's Anatomy* for Franklin to study, and informed Franklin that he would occasionally

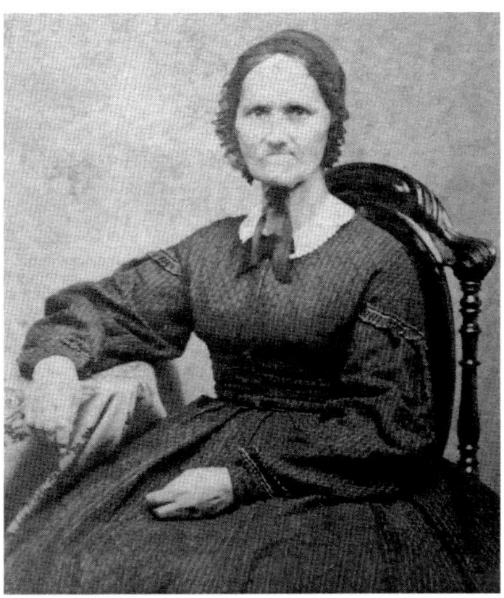

4.4. Grandmother Caroline Martin.

quiz him to make sure that he was making significant progress in learning anatomy. Franklin essentially memorized the text and answered Dr. Spalding's questions in minute detail. Spalding was amazed. It is apparent that Franklin had benefited from his studies at the Elroy Seminary and had learned the discipline necessary to master a complex subject in depth. Spalding next brought out *Gray's Anatomy*, and Franklin repeated his feat. Dr. Spalding gave Franklin his extra copy of *Gray's Anatomy* and advised him not to simply read about anatomy or any other medical subject but to learn and understand the subject in detail. Franklin thought this was some of the best advice a preceptor could give a student of medicine, and he followed that advice throughout his medical studies. Dr. Spalding was a learned man and an excellent mentor. He was well-read and had an astute intellect. Franklin later reflected that his time with Dr. Spalding had taught him intellectual discipline and that the experience was as valuable as any university course.[5]

PLANS FOR MEDICAL SCHOOL IN CHICAGO

While studying under Dr. Spalding, Franklin met Frederick Parkhurst, who was doing a medical preceptorship with Dr. William Whyte, another Watertown physician. Parkhurst, who was more prominent socially than

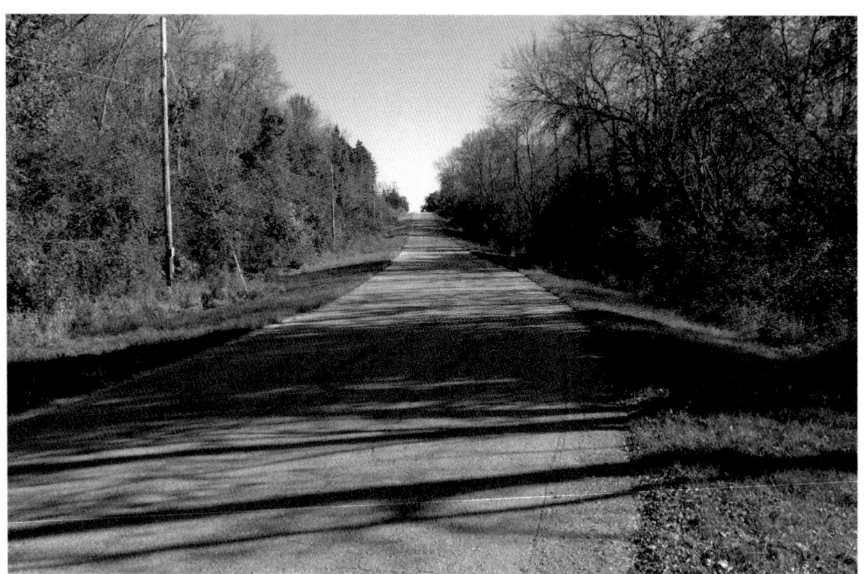

4.5. Branch Road in Ixonia today, where it traverses what was the Martin homestead.

Franklin, wanted him to join his social circle. A friendship slowly developed, and Parkhurst suggested they attend medical school together in Chicago, IL, the following winter. Franklin agreed and they began to plan.

Franklin needed to find employment to raise funds for medical school, now that his six-month preceptorship was complete. But first he needed to help on the family farm.[6] His mother and stepfather had moved to the Munger farm adjacent to the original Martin homestead on the Rock River. He worked there for a short time, but to raise funds for medical school he began working on his Uncle William Fulmer's farm harvesting hay, planting corn and potatoes, and caring for the hops. As had always been true for Franklin, he enjoyed working and socializing with the hospitable Fulmer family. His grandmother Caroline Martin (Figure 4.4) lived with the Fulmers at that time, and although close to 80 years old, she was still in good health and had a sharp mind.

After the fall harvest, Franklin returned to working at the brickyard until it was time to prepare to leave for Chicago. He asked for and received a $25 loan from his Grandmother Martin, as he didn't have the required finances for his first year of medical school—approximately $200.[7]

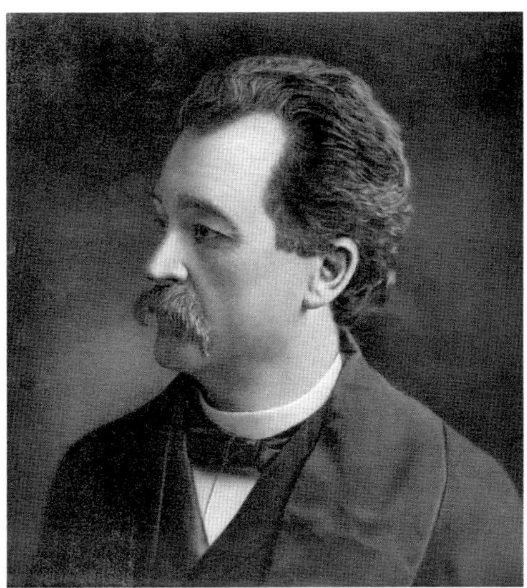

4.6. Dr. Nicholas Senn, another famous Chicago surgeon from Wisconsin.

As the time approached for Franklin to depart, he returned to his parents' home in Ixonia and packed the provisions he would need for life in Chicago. He described in some detail how the wagon trip from the family farm passed through the neighborhood where he grew up (Figure 4.5), with all its familiar, significant surroundings. They drove down Munger Hill, by the site of his parents' first home, and past Grandfather Martin's original log home. They traveled along the big bend in the Rock River, where his Grandfather Carlin and his family had camped on their first night in the area. They passed the Ixonia town center, where the family had first heard of his father's death.

He thought about the impact on his family of his new adventure and reminisced on his time in the lake country of Wisconsin, where he had worked and played for 20 years. He believed that his life in Wisconsin had left him with a strong body and a clear mind. Later, when describing what it was like to leave his beloved lake country, he wrote again of the joy that it brought to him and his anticipation that he would find equal happiness in his future: "Our young souls were filled with joy; and this joy of living was enhanced by anticipation of the immediate future, which, though obscured by inexperience, had the glamour of radiant hopes."[8]

Before leaving, Martin and Parkhurst needed to obtain credentials from the board of censors of the Wisconsin State Medical Society, which would establish their eligibility to become medical school students. These credentials required the signature of Nicholas Senn, MD (Figure 4.6), who later became a respected Chicago surgeon. Dr. Senn recommended that they attend Chicago Medical College (later Northwestern University Medical School). With their certificates signed, they left for Chicago to follow Senn's advice and enroll at Chicago Medical College.[9]

References

1. Martin, F. H. (1933). *The Joy of Living: An Autobiography,* vol. 1 (pp. 115-116). New York, NY: Doubleday, Doran & Co.
2. Ibid., pp. 116-117.
3. Ibid., pp. 117-118.
4. Ibid., pp. 118-119.
5. Ibid., pp. 119-121.
6. Ibid., p. 124.
7. Ibid., pp. 124-126.
8. Ibid., pp. 126-128.
9. Ibid., pp. 128-130.

Chapter 5

Medical School and Internship

oon noised ab ~~—~~ thought t

that the Corlins those had brought h

decisions on Sunday had. Every boo

claim on the big land.

the raising on Saturday. Volunteers

~~hands~~ were busy from all the neig

the week, felling trees, [and] hewing ~~the~~ [addition]

to shape for the new house. Early

g of Saturday a dozen or more stu

and boys were on hand to constru

house. A cellar had been dug in th

~~fouls~~ ready to be encased with ston

alum logs had been sunk in be

reached a bed of solid clay beneath th

il, lumber had been brought fro

aw mill and a fine lot of dry

been contributed by generous neighbors

er ~~oxen~~ ready to compete with Su

that had been brou

sturdy oxen

neighbors.

Jim Hollis by common cons

of the games

ersman for the day. No time was

all directions came the great logs

iron chains about their necks a

of the faithful oxen cheer

Arrival in Chicago

In late September 1877, Martin and Frederick Parkhurst arrived in Chicago at the unimpressive St. Paul Railroad Station near the sewage-filled Chicago River. For two young men who had spent their early lives surrounded by the clear streams and picturesque lakes of southern Wisconsin, this was an unattractive site. In Martin's words, "The river fairly seethed with filth and steamed with foul odors."[1] They checked their belongings at the railroad station and walked to Michigan Avenue, which at the time was equally unimpressive. Martin described it as resembling "the abandoned backyard of a sordid village."[1] The Illinois Central railroad right-of-way that traversed the shallow waters of Lake Michigan tarnished the view from Michigan Avenue. They walked to the Palmer House Hotel which, despite the surrounding blights on the landscape, was still the imposing edifice they expected.

From there they traveled west by mule-drawn streetcar, through areas ravaged by the great Chicago Fire of 1871, to Wood and Harrison Streets, the site of Rush Medical College. It was an impressive building, and they were greeted graciously by college officials and a few enthusiastic students, but they were still convinced that they should attend Chicago Medical College.

They then traveled south to the site of Chicago Medical College at 26th Street and Prairie Avenue, and saw an undistinguished, old, and battered building with bare, dusty walls and neglected floors. No officials or enthusiastic students welcomed them. A janitor showed them the two amphitheaters, the museum where they saw the mounted skeleton of "Jumbo" the circus elephant, and the chemical laboratory. After a short tour, they met with two college instructors who acted as guides and assured them that despite the older buildings, Chicago Medical College had fewer but better-quality students than Rush. It had a three-year rather than a two-year curriculum, a relationship with nearby Mercy Hospital, and a high-quality faculty. Martin and Parkhurst were

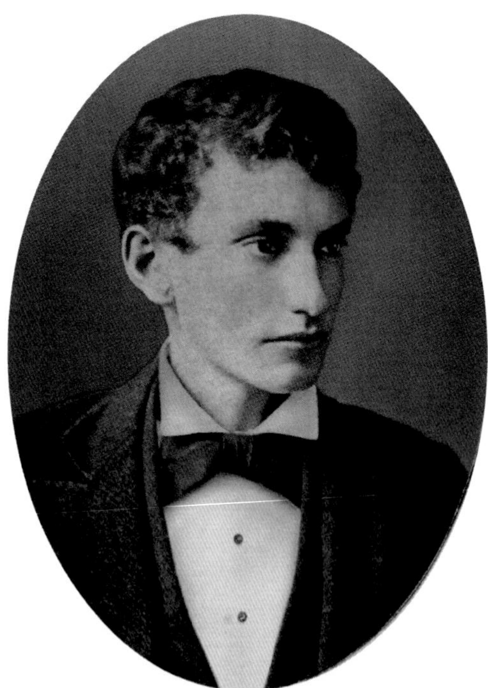

5.1. Franklin Martin, circa the time he left for medical school in Chicago.

impressed and left immediately to register for classes with Dr. Daniel Nelson, faculty registrar. After Dr. Nelson advised them not to carry large amounts of money in a big city like Chicago, they called on the school treasurer, Dr. Hollister, and paid their first year's tuition.

Next, they needed to find a place to live. After a long search, they located rooms they could afford at 1133 State Street. The partially furnished apartment was better than they'd expected and adequate for their needs, but not nearly as grand as the apartments of many of their wealthier classmates. The apartment had one small sleeping room with a double bed, a larger room with a table and chairs, and a sink with running water in the hall. The landlady agreed to a price of $4 a month if they would furnish the larger room, which they agreed to do.

In short order, they retrieved their belongings from the train station and unpacked. To prepare their meals they purchased a cookstove and utensils from a local secondhand store. That first evening they dined on a fine meal:

> The supper consisted of baked potatoes, savory salt pork that floated in its own brown fat, bread transported from our Wisconsin farm, butter churned by Mother, preserves from the wild plums along the Rock River, fruits and nuts. The above menu was generously amplified by the cakes, pies, and doughnuts which had been fitted into the corners of our two trunks.[1]

They were quite pleased with all they had accomplished their first day in Chicago and slept well that night in their comfortable bed. With rent of only $1 a week, the food they had brought from home supplemented by small purchases from the local grocery, and only minor additional expenses, they still had some money for incidentals. They were adapting quickly to big city life.

Martin and Parkhurst filled their free days before the term started exploring the college buildings and observing the other students who were enrolling. They consulted college representatives about what to expect once classes began and where to purchase secondhand textbooks.

Just before classes commenced, they had an opportunity to watch Dr. Edmund Andrews perform a leg amputation. Dr. Andrews was a favorite among the students and received uproarious applause upon entering the old, large, tiered-seat amphitheater at Mercy Hospital. Dr. Andrews was one of the first surgeons in the Midwest to use the English surgeon Sir Joseph Lister's antiseptic techniques during surgical procedures. In addition, he was a strong supporter of Lister among his fellow surgeons.[2] The use of antiseptics during operative procedures was not the standard of care at that time in the U.S. and instead was openly ridiculed by many prominent Americans surgeons, even though it was becoming the standard of care in many areas of Europe.[3] Exposure to the use of antiseptics in the operating room at this early stage of his medical education had a major impact on Martin.

An intern performed the anesthesia using an ether-saturated towel placed over the patient's face. Fumes filled the amphitheater, giving many of the students their first opportunity to inhale ether. The surgical instruments were soaked in a 5 percent solution of carbolic acid (phenol) to render them antiseptic. The surgeon soaked his hands in 2½ percent carbolic acid, and the patient's leg also was washed with the solution. The use of carbolic acid as an antiseptic in the operating room at that time was not the standard of care. A tourniquet was placed above the site of the proposed amputation to control bleeding. With a long-bladed amputation knife, the surgeon cut the flesh through to the bone in two strokes and then amputated the leg using a bone saw. Large vessels were tied with silk suture and the tourniquet removed. The wound was then closed with silk sutures and covered with a dressing of cotton soaked in 5 percent carbolized oil. In Martin's words, "It was our baptism of blood."[1]

FIRST YEAR OF MEDICAL SCHOOL

On October 1, 1877, Martin (Figure 5.1), age 20, started classes at the Chicago Medical College (Figure 5.2). The Dean of Chicago Medical College, the dignified and distinguished Dr. Nathan Smith Davis, greeted them at the student gathering that opened the school year. Martin said of Dr. Davis, "His strong character attracted, his earnestness and seriousness of purpose compelled, and his logic inspired."[4]

In their first year, the students would study descriptive anatomy, physiology, histology, inorganic chemistry, materia medica (pharmacology), dissections, the use of the microscope, and practical work in the chemical laboratory. Each of their professors gave the impression that the subject they were teaching must be mastered as though it was the most important class in the curriculum. In view of this opinion, Martin and Parkhurst decided that they could make up for what they believed was their inadequate previous education by working hard and completing each day's assignments before retiring; they wanted to start each day with their coursework up to date. Martin later asserted that making that decision at the beginning of his medical studies was essential to his success. He and Parkhurst realized the seriousness of the responsibility to study hard, but they thought that their backgrounds and work ethic gave them unlimited capacity to succeed despite the lack of a formal undergraduate education. This attitude is reminiscent of the mindset Franklin developed when he worked in the fields and the brickyard. The two students decided that the only relaxation they would routinely allow themselves was to take daily walks around Chicago. They also decided they would eat wholesome meals to stay fit and healthy.

Because of their dedication to their studies and their avoidance of social functions, the two men performed well, while many of their col-

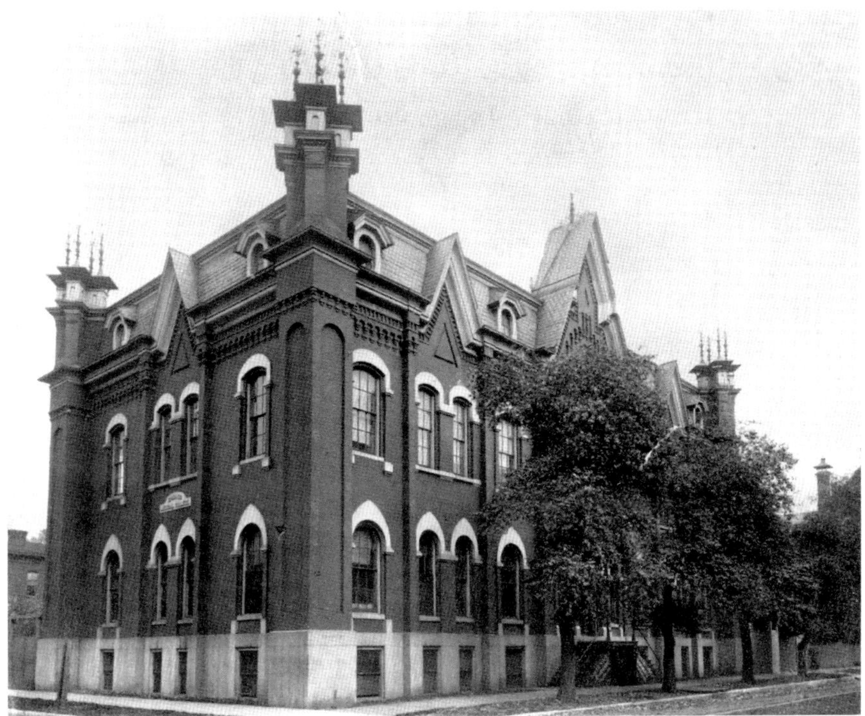

5.2. Chicago Medical College (26th Street and Prairie Avenue) circa 1880, when Martin was a student.

leagues did not. As the first year continued, they had to increase the intensity of their studies to have any chance of being in the group of successful students at the end of the school year. Because they adhered strictly to their study schedule, they developed only a few friendships.

The young men were just able to meet their financial obligations, but a problem arose because their landlord insisted that they pay the rent on time. In December, under the threat of eviction because they were unable to pay their rent on the stipulated day, they had to seek an emergency loan from a friend. Otherwise, because of the food supplies sent from home, they were able to support themselves and remain well fed.

Martin and Parkhurst were uneasy about allowing their few friends to see their meager apartment and went to great lengths to avoid having guests, which only made their acquaintances more curious. One evening a classmate, John Mulholland, walking with Martin, refused to leave until Martin took him to the apartment. Once there, Mulholland thoroughly enjoyed himself and put Martin and Parkhurst at ease. They began inviting other classmates to their home for coffee and cookies and doughnuts from Wisconsin. Much to their relief, such events genuinely appealed to their colleagues. With this new openness, they began coaching a few classmates who had fallen behind in their studies. Martin and Parkhurst continued their own solid academic performance and passed their examinations at the end of the first year, along with all their friends.

At the end of the school year, it was time to return to Wisconsin to work for funds to continue their schooling. Parkhurst was to teach at a district school back in Wisconsin. Martin decided that returning to work in his Uncle George Fulmer's brickyard would be more lucrative and wrote to his uncle, who assented. They packed up and stored their household goods and furniture in a college building under the care of the janitor and returned to Wisconsin.[4]

Making Bricks Again

Martin felt privileged to have the opportunity to return to work alongside his Fulmer cousins and "to enjoy life in an environment of honest, God-fearing people who were full of the joy of living."[5] He admired his cousins and people like them who believed work was a necessary part of life and that no man should shirk his daily task. His cousins worked long, hard days but were always ready to relax in the evening.

At this time Martin was becoming more social. In addition to his favorite recreational activities of fishing, hunting, baseball, picnics, and visiting friends and family, there was buggy riding in the company of young ladies along the country and village roads of Wisconsin's lake country, and on rare occasions dancing. But Martin still felt a bit shy. One day, an attractive young lady from a nearby resort stopped to watch him emptying bricks from the molds; she praised him for the straightness of his artistically placed rows of bricks. She asked to be allowed to carry one of the molds. Martin found a leather apron like the one he wore and placed it on her. She then carried the 40-pound mold the length of the yard and with Martin's assistance placed it on its side, which required that Martin stand close behind her to guide her. Martin concluded his description of the episode, "The personality of this little 'tomboy' maiden gave a genuine thrill to as many of my

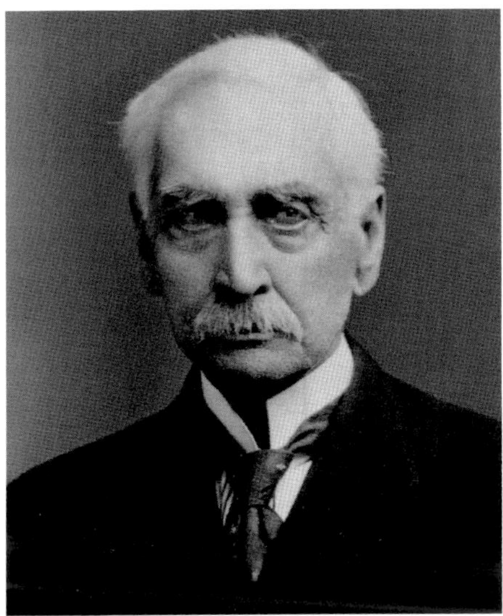

5.3. Uncle Addison Carlin, Martin's supportive uncle who assisted him financially during medical school.

youthful fellow workers as could discreetly watch the performance from a distance, and it was food for many hours of dreams."[5]

UNCLE "AD" HELPS

Martin needed additional funds for the second year of medical school, more than he could possibly earn working in the brickyard, so he appealed to his uncle Addison Carlin (Figure 5.3), who had become wealthy prospecting for gold in Montana and the Black Hills of South Dakota. On returning to Watertown, Uncle "Ad" wisely invested a large sum in farm mortgages, which substantially increased his wealth. He kept some of the gold bricks at home where, family legend had it, Aunt Mary placed the gold in woolen sacks to disguise them and used them as doorstops around the house.

Uncle Ad had always been generous, but Martin was still nervous about approaching him with a request for substantial funds. He composed a letter to Uncle Ad outlining his financial needs for the next two years of school and how his summer wages would be insufficient. In reply, Uncle Ad asked that Martin come to Watertown for a weekend to discuss his finances. After a meeting, not only did Uncle Ad give him enough money for another year of school, he also bought Martin a completely new wardrobe, which he sorely needed. Uncle Ad did not expect to be repaid, but Martin insisted that he accept a promissory note that he intended to repay. It is obvious why a family member, William Cubbins, said, "Aunt Mary and Uncle Addison Carlin were a dominating influence for good in his life."[6] On Franklin's return to the Munger farm, his mother reminded him in no uncertain terms of the importance of repaying Uncle Ad with his initial earnings after he became a doctor.[7]

Second Year of Medical School

On arrival in Chicago for the second year of medical school, Martin and Parkhurst discovered that the college janitor who had agreed to store their household goods at the college was no longer employed by the school, and their goods were gone. In addition, their apartment had been rented to someone else. After a short search, they found a new room on 25th Street, one-and-a-half blocks from the college. Unlike their old abode, this apartment had no separate bedroom and was unfurnished. Although the men were disappointed in the new space, the more pressing problem was the unplanned expense of purchasing new furnishings and household goods.[8]

Martin and Parkhurst were prepared for the intensity of their second-year studies and even enjoyed the return to their routine. Again, they studied long hours, and they began a new practice of frequently quizzing each other. These quiz sessions often led to disagreements. Parkhurst's answers were taken verbatim from the book, whereas Martin would give an equally correct answer using his own words. The arguments often were intense, resulting in an abrupt end to the session. To Martin's chagrin, Parkhurst became too focused in his approach to his coursework and refused to go on the evening walks that were rejuvenating for Martin, who would go out on his own. He said, "These walks gave me great pleasure, and they were unsurpassed as uplifters of my spirits."[9]

Martin and Parkhurst's social status had improved to the point that their one-room apartment became a gathering place for many of their classmates. These visits frequently developed into tutoring sessions.

Uncle Addison came to Chicago and treated Martin and Parkhurst to dinner at the Palmer House Hotel, after which they went to see a play. The following day they took Uncle Ad on a tour of the medical school, which he thoroughly enjoyed. It became obvious to Martin that the real purpose of Uncle Ad's visit to Chicago was to casually observe Martin in his new surroundings. Martin felt it was difficult for his family in Wisconsin to believe that something constructive could come from anything except hard physical labor. The visit appeared to change Uncle Ad's viewpoint and left him with the impression that Martin's endeavors were worthwhile.

Martin and Parkhurst's diligence during the first year of medical school paid off. It gave them a solid foundation, making their second-year coursework much easier to comprehend. The subjects that year were more practical, and the importance of learning the basics of anatomy, physiology, chemistry, and other subjects became obvious. They passed their end-of-year examinations without difficulty and returned to Wisconsin for the summer.[9]

TEACHING AT OAK GROVE SCHOOL

With Parkhurst's assistance, Martin obtained a post for the summer of 1879 as teacher for the upper grades at the Oak Grove School in Wisconsin; but he needed a teacher certificate for Dodge County. He passed a special examination with the superintendent of schools and received the certificate. The Oak Grove School was 17 miles north of Watertown (Figure 5.4). To get to Oak Grove, Martin first took a train to the nearby town of Juneau and walked, to save money and enjoy the countryside, the last three miles to his destination. He arrived at the Oak Grove Hotel, which he found charming but knew was beyond his means. The gentleman proprietor, Mr. Griffin, kindly told him to pay whatever he could afford until he found another place. Mrs. Griffin also welcomed him as though he were "a distinguished guest, worthy to become a member of the family."[10] A week later, Martin began his search for an affordable boardinghouse, but the Griffins had become fond of him and said they would be delighted if he would continue to stay with them and only pay what he could afford. He was grateful and happy to be accepted "to live for two months in that paradise" by people he admired.

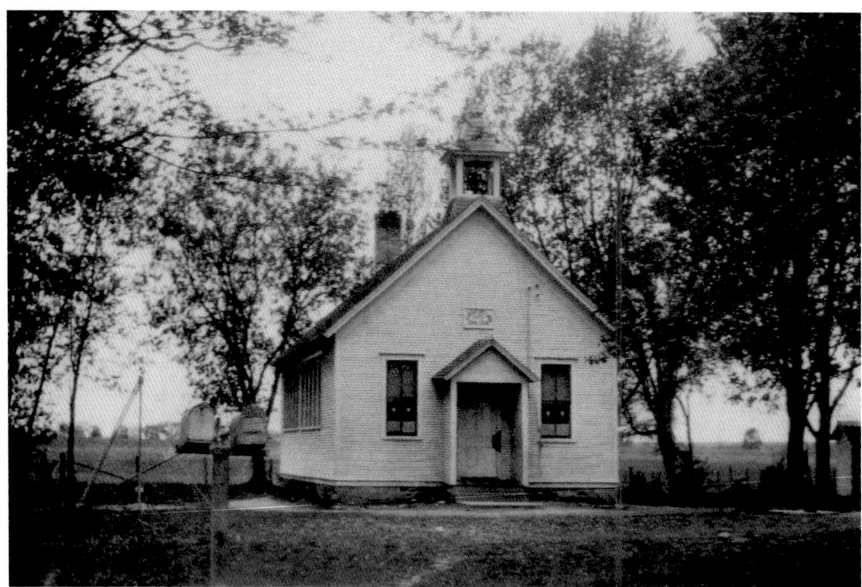

5.4. Oak Grove School, Oak Grove, WI, where Martin taught.

Martin was a dedicated teacher who put tremendous energy into his work. He divided the students into three grades and assigned them specific tasks. They were to memorize and recite passages from select literary classics. He used somewhat original teaching methods; for example, in addition to recitations and several pages of reading, the students were to work out mathematical problems in detail and be prepared to display the results on the blackboard. The following day, none of the students had completed the assignment. He gave them additional time to work but told them that if they could not complete the assignment, he would work with them on it. Despite the long hours of study required and the intense classroom discussions, the students came to accept Martin's methods, and they developed a mutual respect.

He believed it was a successful summer. He had encountered refined people and had the satisfaction of knowing that he had become friends with many of them, despite his persistent feeling that he was a poor conversationalist and ill at ease around strangers. He thought his inexperience in life, his original teaching methods, his energy, and his love of sports made him a curiosity.[10]

Third Year of Medical School

Martin and Parkhurst returned to the same apartment and prepared for their third and final year of medical school, which began September 30, 1879. Martin had the money he had earned over the summer plus an additional $150 loan from Uncle Ad. As they had done in past years, the family provided a plentiful supply of food, including an abundance of his mother's jams, jellies, and preserves. As they continued their routine of hard work, a wholesome diet, and daily exercise, Martin and Parkhurst found their third-year studies much easier. Martin again attributed this to their disciplined approach to their studies in the first two years. This term was more enjoyable because of the genuine friendship and companionship of a small cadre of classmates.

The teachers for the third-year curriculum were well-known Chicago medical practitioners with citywide reputations. Martin later indicated that at that time the "art of medicine" as opposed to the "science of medicine" was taught in medical school, but the science was being developed and would pair with the art in the future.[11] Martin's belief in the importance of the science of medicine is demonstrated by his dedication to volume 2 of his autobiography: "To My Friend THE SCIENTIFICALLY TRAINED DOCTOR who with honesty and industry serves men, women, and little children by preserving their health and curing their ills; and who strives to maintain the sanctity and independence of the scientific profession of medicine."[12]

Martin and Parkhurst continued their solid performance and again generously invited other students to practice sessions in their apartment. During these sessions, they discussed likely final examination questions. Many of the students who attended these evenings were poor readers who did not always grasp the information in a textbook but were more likely to comprehend the concepts presented in discussions. In the end, Martin, Parkhurst, and all but one of the other study group members passed their final examinations and became physicians.[11]

Applying for Internship Positions

Toward the end of the third year of school, there were competitive examinations and interviews for internship positions. Twenty-four internship positions were available at Cook County Hospital in

Chicago, all of which were filled by students from Chicago Medical College and Rush Medical College. For unclear reasons, Martin and Parkhurst were not candidates for the Cook County Hospital internship positions. Medical students from both schools were permitted to observe the examinations and interviews for the internships. It was in these interviews that Martin first encountered Dr. John B. Murphy and he, along with many other students, was impressed with how well Dr. Murphy performed. Later Murphy became an accomplished and respected Chicago surgeon who invented the Murphy button for performing intestinal anastomoses without sutures. He and Martin went on to become great friends and collaborators.

Parkhurst and Martin were invited to be candidates for the two internship positions at Mercy Hospital in Chicago, and at first it appeared that they would be the only candidates. After Martin had completed his examination and Parkhurst had begun his, Martin, believing that no other students were vying for the positions, freely discussed the questions and his answers. After Parkhurst exited the room, one of their classmates and friends, Lorenzo T. Potter, announced that he wanted to interview for the position. After a short conversation with Parkhurst about the questions he had been asked, Martin realized that they both had been asked identical questions, and so Potter had the advantage of having heard Martin discuss the answers. In addition, Potter was one of the students that Martin and Parkhurst had coached during the school year, so Martin knew that he could give clear answers. The examiners ranked Potter first, Martin second, and Parkhurst third, much to Martin's consternation. Martin obtained an internship position, but Parkhurst did not. As a result, Parkhurst elected to accept a position as an associate of his uncle, Dr. Harvey Parkhurst, a practitioner in Danvers, IL.[13]

Graduation

On March 3, 1880, Martin graduated and received his medical degree at Plymouth Church, 26th Street and Michigan Avenue. In front of a large audience that regrettably did not include any of his family, he and his classmates marched down the center aisle of the church and were presented with their diplomas.[14]

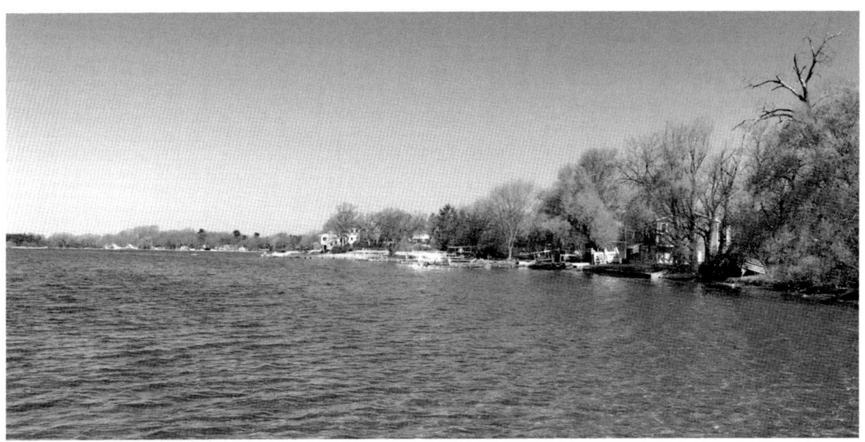

5.5. Recent photograph of the Silver Lake area, where Martin's mother Josephine, his stepfather Elon Munger, and sister Jeanette lived in the 1870s and 1880s and where Martin spent a month relaxing before returning to Chicago to begin his internship.

POSITION CARING FOR WILLIAM HICKLING

Martin's internship position did not open for six months, and he was without funds to support himself in the interim. Luckily, at the last minute, a medical school professor recommended Martin for a post caring for a wealthy, educated, elderly man, William Hickling, at $5 a day plus room and board. This was more than double the pay he would have received if he had returned to Wisconsin to work in the brickyard. He happily accepted the six-month situation. The work was not challenging, but it gave him the opportunity to meet several interesting and powerful people. He had time to read and discuss the classics and talk about politics with Mr. Hickling and his friends. He even had an opportunity to attend the 1880 Republican convention because of the generosity of one of Mr. Hickling's acquaintances. Martin, because of his Grandfather Carlin's interest in national politics, developed a lifelong interest in the national political scene and was thrilled to have the chance to attend the convention where James A. Garfield was nominated for President on the thirty-fifth ballot. His interest in politics certainly helps explain why he was thrilled when he had the opportunity to work within the government in the nation's preparation for entry into World War I. Attending the convention was an experience through which Martin grew intellectually and one he appreciated his whole life.

The most significant outcome from this employment was that, to his great satisfaction, he was able to repay the loans from Grandmother Martin and Uncle Addison Carlin. Toward the end of Martin's time as caregiver, Mr. Hickling's physician, Dr. Edmund Andrews, noted that Martin was thin and pale and recommended that he take a vacation and get some sunshine before beginning his internship at Mercy Hospital.[15]

Relaxing with Family Prior to Beginning Internship

Following Dr. Andrews' recommendation, Martin returned to Wisconsin to spend time with his family before his internship. He spent one month relaxing with his mother, stepfather, and his sister Nettie on their small farm near Silver Lake, south of Oconomowoc (Figure 5.5). It had been a year since he had been able to spend significant amounts of time outdoors exercising and enjoying his surroundings. He fished, explored Silver Lake, relaxed in the sunshine, and walked in the moonlight. He was a happy man with a wonderful future that he was eagerly anticipating. He considered that he had been treated as a distinguished guest and a beloved member of a happy family. He said, "Color came to my faded cheeks, strength to my unused muscles, and flesh to my lean body."[16] The happy month left him with tender memories of his wholesome life in Wisconsin, but it was time to return to Chicago to begin his internship and his medical career.[16] Except for trips to conduct family business, he did not return to Wisconsin for almost 20 years.

Even as the years went by, the lifestyle and surroundings that his family and friends enjoyed in the lake country of southern Wisconsin would most certainly have continued to stand in harsh contrast to his lifestyle and surroundings in Chicago. Even today, rural life in the wonderful landscape of Wisconsin lake country contrasts sharply with the environment of big cities—to which anyone who has lived in both environs can attest.

Internship at Mercy Hospital

In the fall of 1880, Martin returned to the now-familiar Chicago to begin his internship at the well-known Mercy Hospital at 26th Street and Calumet Avenue (Figure 5.6). On arrival at the facility, he was

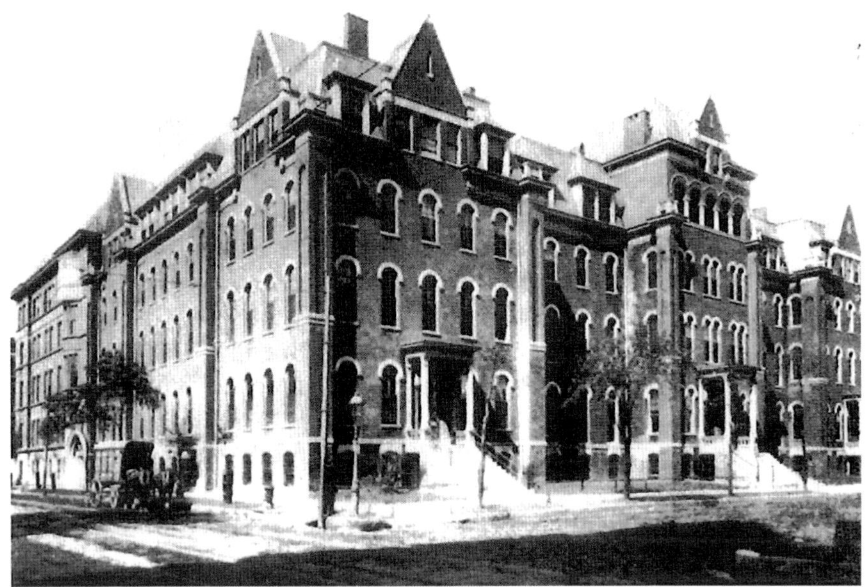

5.6. Mercy Hospital (26th Street and Calumet Avenue) circa 1880, when Martin did his internship.

greeted by Sister Raphael, who went on to become famous as the hospital's executive. There were comfortable living quarters with good lighting, a nice bed, and a private dining room that served high-quality food. His friend and the senior intern, Dr. Lorenzo Potter, took him on a tour and introduced him to one of his main responsibilities, the dressing of wounds.

At this time, medicine and surgery were undergoing the transition from the "pre-germ theory" era to an era when the methods of clinical practice would be highly influenced by the concepts of bacteriology. There was bitter controversy over the theory that bacteria were the cause of many diseases, both surgical and nonsurgical. In 1865, the surgeon Sir Joseph Lister, after reading Louis Pasteur's earlier work on the subject, became convinced that bacteria were responsible for surgical wound infections. After studying various methods to protect wounds from bacterial contamination, Lister decided to use carbolic acid. In his initial studies with the use of carbolic acid in 1865, Lister treated patients with compound fractures (bone fractures where the bone punctures the skin). At this time compound fractures frequently became infected and resulted in amputations. In his study patients' wounds were irrigated with a carbolic acid solution, and the wounds covered with a dressing soaked in carbolic acid. Over the next few days, carbolic acid was reapplied to the wounds multiple times daily. Of the nine compound fractures that Lister treated in this manner, eight recovered without amputation, resulting in a failure rate of only 11 percent. These results were very encouraging to Lister and he proceeded with a new study on the treatment of abscesses.[17]

When treating abscesses, Lister first irrigated the abscess cavity with carbolic acid and then placed a carbolic acid-soaked dressing in the cavity. Another carbolic acid-soaked dressing was placed over this. Most of the abscesses healed without complications. Lister said, "[The]course run by cases of abscesses treated in this way is so *beautifully* in harmony with the theory of the whole subject of suppuration…."[18]

In his early studies of the use of antiseptics during operations, Lister soaked the instruments in carbolic acid. Also, the surgeons dipped their hands in a similar solution and it was applied to the surgical site.[19] After the operation, the wound was covered with gauze soaked in a solution of carbolic acid. This protocol significantly reduced the wound infection rate. The mortality rate on Lister's wards decreased from 45 percent in the period prior to initiating the carbolic acid protocol to 15 percent afterward. It wasn't until 1871 that Lister began using the atomizer to spray carbolic acid into the air in the operating room, because he believed air was one source of bacterial contamination of surgical wounds.[20] Regrettably, because of its unusual appearance, many people believe that Lister's only contribution to operating room antisepsis was the atomizer.

Many respected physicians were adamantly opposed to, and ridiculed, the germ theory of diseases. Others openly accepted the possibility that bacteria could cause disease. Martin believed it was important that physicians have an open mind about the topic, and slowly he came to believe that the bacteriologists were correct, although it wasn't until after 1890 that the germ theory of postoperative wound infections was more universally accepted in the U.S. By 1900, almost all operations were performed using appropriate precautions, but even at that time there were some skeptics.

On his daily dressing rounds, Martin, as did all interns, carried a wooden tray with five compartments containing the supplies necessary to dress patients' wounds. Many of the wounds were horrific, and it was extremely painful for the patients to have them cleaned and dressed. The experience of carrying out these procedures had a lasting impact on Martin.

Dressing boxes were a fixture on surgical wards for more than 100 years, until it was discovered that they carried infectious microorganisms from patient to patient. Martin also was upset by the ignorance that perpetuated the preantiseptic era and the impact it had on patients' lives. In 1880, approximately 90 percent of surgical wounds became infected, and a high percentage of patients undergoing abdominal surgery died. In view of these negative results, he was encouraged when the fundamental principles of germ theory began to be integrated into clinical practice.

During Martin's internship two major epidemics occurred in Chicago that affected his training experience. The first was a typhoid fever epidemic, a disease for which at that time there was no proven treatment. In a high percentage of patients, the disease would reach a crisis when the fever would peak and then slowly abate. Some patients would collapse and die, and some would die of intestinal hemorrhage or perforation. The epidemic went on for many weeks, during which time numerous patients were admitted to the hospital. The exhausting routine of caring for these acutely ill patients was stressful and wearing on the strength and morale of the staff, not unlike what has occurred more recently with the coronavirus disease 2019 pandemic.

An epidemic of smallpox developed as the typhoid fever epidemic was subsiding. Because of the efforts of an Englishman, Dr. Edward Jenner, for a century there had been an efficacious vaccine against smallpox; regrettably, it was not universally in use. The epidemic spread rapidly throughout the city of Chicago, overwhelming the health care system. Hospitals and pesthouses were filled beyond capacity. A program was begun to vaccinate as many people as possible. In Martin's experience, no one who had been properly vaccinated developed a severe case of smallpox.

Both epidemics had a significant impact on Martin. Obviously he was upset by the suffering and death he observed with smallpox, despite the fact that it was essentially a preventable disease. He was critical of the people who ridiculed the smallpox vaccination and called them ignorant and unthinking.[21]

Time to Plan for the Future

With his internship completed, it was time for Martin to begin making plans for his future. He had a keen interest in the research being conducted on antiseptic surgery and specifically the work of Dr. Edward W. Jenks, a noted Detroit gynecologist, who had recently been appointed to the staff of Chicago's Mercy Hospital. Soon after Dr. Jenks started practicing gynecology at the hospital in 1881, he made plans to perform an operation using antiseptic surgery. Martin was invited to be the anesthetist for the operation.

In his autobiography, Martin described in detail the operation and postoperative course of the patient, who was having an oophorectomy for a large ovarian tumor. As was then the protocol for performing antiseptic surgery, the room was sprayed with carbolic acid in the days prior to the operation. On the day of the operation, the room was again saturated with spray from the carbolic acid atomizer. Just before making the incision the abdominal wall was prepped with carbolic acid and all other elements of Lister's antisepsis protocol completed. The abdomen was opened using a midline incision, and with minimal problems the tumor was removed. The wound was closed with through-and-through sutures. The postoperative course was uneventful. There was no "laudable pus." On postoperative day 10, the dressing was removed, the skin sponged with carbolic acid solution, and the stitches removed. Many of the physicians present had never seen an abdominal wound that had healed without signs of infection. Martin was impressed and intrigued by the impact that Lister's theories on antiseptic surgery was having on the care and lives of patients.[22]

Because of his experience working with Dr. Jenks and his review of the medical literature, Martin decided to apply antiseptic techniques to the care of patients on the obstetrical ward. Before examining patients, he dipped his hands in carbolic acid and bathed the patient's perineum with the same solution. None of the first 75 patients he cared for on the obstetrical ward using this procedure died from infection, and none developed childbed (puerperal) fever. With this experience he became an enthusiastic supporter of Lister's theory of antisepsis. It is amazing that at such an early stage in his career he grasped the implications of the germ theory of infection and designed a protocol to help prevent puerperal fever, which occurred at a very high rate in postpartum women. Prior to this others, including Dr. Ignaz Semmelweis, had advocated for handwashing and the washing of caregivers' apparel after contact with infected patients on the obstetrical wards; but Martin's use of an antiseptic to control the spread of puerperal fever was unique.

Based on these and similar experiences, Martin developed an interest in obstetrics and gynecology, and when offered a position in the department of gynecology and the diseases of women at the South Side Dispensary, he enthusiastically accepted.[23]

REFERENCES

1. Martin, F. H. (1933). *The Joy of Living: An Autobiography,* vol. 1 (pp. 130-139). New York, NY: Doubleday, Doran & Co.
2. Rutkow, I. M. (1988). *The History of Surgery in the United States: 1775-1900* (pp. 373-374). San Francisco, CA: Norman Publishing, Jeremy Norman & Co.
3. Fitzharris, L. (2017). *The Butchering Art: Joseph Lister's Quest to Transform the Grisly World of Victorian Medicine* (pp. 214-223). New York, NY: Scientific American, Farrar, Strauss and Giroux.
4. Ibid., pp. 140-148.
5. Ibid., pp. 149-150.
6. Cubbins, W. (1935). Franklin H. Martin. *Bull Am Coll Surg,* 20(2), 39.
7. Martin, F. H. (1933). *The Joy of Living: An Autobiography,* vol. 1 (pp. 151-155). New York, NY: Doubleday, Doran & Co.
8. Ibid., p. 156.
9. Ibid., pp. 157-161.
10. Ibid., pp. 161-170.
11. Ibid., pp. 177-180.
12. Martin, F. H. (1933). *The Joy of Living: An Autobiography,* vol. 2 (dedication page). New York, NY: Doubleday, Doran & Co.
13. Martin, F. H. (1933). *The Joy of Living: An Autobiography,* vol. 1 (pp. 180-182). New York, NY: Doubleday, Doran & Co.
14. Ibid., pp. 188-189.
15. Ibid., pp. 185-195.
16. Ibid., p. 196.

17. Fitzharris, L. (2017). *The Butchering Art: Joseph Lister's Quest to Transform the Grisly World of Victorian Medicine* (pp. 161-167). New York, NY: Scientific American, Farrar, Strauss and Giroux.
18. Ibid., p. 168.
19. Ibid., p. 199.
20. Ibid., pp. 208-210.
21. Martin, F. H. (1933). *The Joy of Living: An Autobiography,* vol.1 (pp. 197-207). New York, NY: Doubleday, Doran & Co.
22. Ibid., pp. 208-213.
23. Ibid., pp. 214-216.

Chapter 6

Getting Established

oon noised ab those ~~was~~ thought t
that the Corliss those had brought
Sessions on Sunday had. Every boo
claim on the big bend.
the raising on Saturday. Volunteer
~~hands~~ were busy from all the neig
additio
and
the week, felling trees, hewing ~~the~~
to shape for the new house. Early
g of Saturday a dozen or more sti
nd boys were on hand to construc
house. ~~A~~ cellar had been dug in t
~~...~~ ready to be encased with sto
ation logs had been sunk in tren
eached a bed of solid clay beneath th
il, lumber had been brought from
aw mill and a fine lot of dry o
been contributed by generous neighbors
en ~~...~~ ready to compete with se
sturdy oxen that had been brou
neighbors.

By mutual common cons
of the game
woman for the day. No time was
all directions came the great logs
iron chains about their necks a
of the faithful oxen

Exploring Minneapolis as a Site to Begin Practicing Medicine

Initially Martin decided to begin practicing medicine in Minneapolis, MN, where as a teenager he had worked as an apprentice millwright in his Uncle Adolphus Guilder's flour mill and manufacturing plant. He believed that his cousin and dear friend Ella Guilder would be helpful to him as he established his practice. Ella was head of her father's household and had influential friends in Minneapolis. Martin traveled to Minneapolis to survey the city and seek a location for an office. He felt received as a prodigal son and was warmly welcomed by Ella and Uncle Adolphus, both of whom encouraged him to establish his medical practice there. He found an acceptable location for his office and went so far as to pay a month's rent. Ella was especially eager to help him get established.[1]

A Chance to Practice Medicine at Mercy Hospital as a Senior Intern

When the Mercy Hospital gynecologist, Dr. Edward W. Jenks, became ill with debilitating hay fever and had to leave Chicago until fall, Martin, still a senior intern, was given the opportunity to step in as attending physician for Dr. Jenks' patients. He was thrilled by the new responsibility of caring for patients without a supervising physician to review his diagnosis and care plans. The experience stimulated him to formulate many questions about women's health, especially conditions that resulted in chronic pain and lethargy. Examples of questions he posed were: "Why were our women semi-invalids, and their male companions healthy and strong?" "Why did they consistently complain of backache, of dragging, and of pelvic weakness?" "Why the exhaustion, and the anemic appearance?" "Why were they unable to enjoy long walks or any form of physical activity?"[2] He found no concrete diagnoses or treatments in the medical literature for the women's ailments. It is intriguing that he was asking such questions so early in his practice of medicine and at a time when most physicians were not so inclined.

Even without a diagnosis, and likely because of his attentiveness, many of Martin's patients improved, with increased strength and decreased pain; but frequently the syndrome recurred. It continued to bother him that medicine had no diagnoses for their problems. Despite this conundrum, Martin believed that he was developing skill, and he had a reputation among his patients for being a good physician. At this early stage in his career, his thoughtful approach to any problem, however difficult, allowed him to seek and define solutions when others could not. Even at this young age, he had the confidence to move forward once he had what he believed was a satisfactory diagnosis and treatment plan.[2]

A Change of Plans

In Martin's estimation, Chicago, with two medical schools and several hospitals, was becoming a center of high-quality medicine, which caused him to reconsider moving his medical practice to Minneapolis. In Chicago, he already had a small practice, as well as many acquaintances in and outside the medical profession. After extensive consideration, he decided to cancel his Minneapolis lease. Instead, he rented a Chicago office in the Central Hall Building at 22nd Street and Wabash Avenue (Figure 6.1). Many well-known physicians had offices in the building, which was in a fashionable neighborhood—a fact Martin considered important for the growth of his practice. He began taking his meals at a local boardinghouse that he considered "desirable"—another factor important in building his reputation. This strategy was successful, as many of his early patients came from the neighborhood boardinghouses. Overall, his patients did well, and his practice flourished as his satisfied patients spread the word. He was pleased when one of the landladies at his boardinghouse sought out his care. In addition, he found his work at the Chicago Medical College dispensary clinic, where he saw patients and discussed their ailments with medical students, both stimulating and important.[3]

Martin realized that most successful medical practitioners earned the confidence and cooperation of their patients, took an interest in

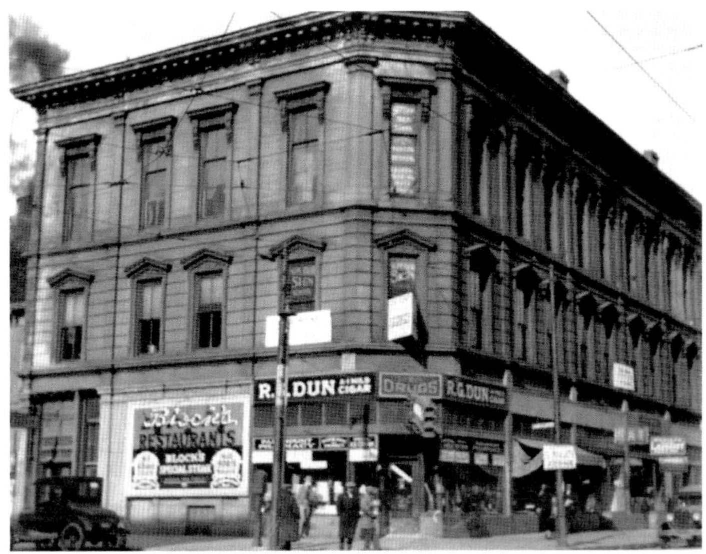

6.1. Central Hall Building (22nd Street and Wabash Avenue), where Martin had his first office, late 1800s.

their patients' illnesses, and discussed the diagnoses and recommended treatment in detail. In his words, "The true practitioner must not be too disinterested, too mechanical nor too academic, and he must have a soul. I was always more deeply interested in my patients and their condition than in anything else, and I endeavored to make the task before me a real game with competitive aims."[4] This description is reminiscent of Martin's description of his Grandfather Carlin's approach to work: "Grandfather made play of work and instilled a spirit of contest in all who worked with him."[5]

By 1882, after practicing for a little more than a year, Martin began to make the acquaintance of several influential families in the Chicago community, who chose him as their family physician and recommended him to their friends. He also cared for local industry managers and workers and their families.[6]

Martin had outlined a multifaceted plan for establishing his medical practice in Chicago, and had achieved almost all the plan's aspects, leading to an increasingly successful medical practice. He evaluated a circumstance and created an effective solution, as he often had done when assigned tasks when working in the fields and the brickyard.

Takes on a Partner

Martin's growing practice and affluent patients attracted the attention of his medical school friend, Dr. Lorenzo Potter, who wanted to join him. Martin was agreeable and took Dr. Potter as a partner. This arrangement meant that Martin could no longer live in his office suite. He and Potter rented a room at the Lords' boardinghouse, at 2225 Wabash Avenue, where Potter became a favorite of the other boarders.[6]

Growing Interest in Gynecology and Obstetrics and Surgery

Slowly his interest in gynecology and obstetrics grew, in part because at that time gynecology included all pelvic and abdominal surgery. In his practice at the South Side Dispensary, Martin had the opportunity to perform minor operations on patients who, because they were indigent, were unable to find care elsewhere. Although he received no remuneration for these services, he sought out the opportunity to perform these operations—many of which were performed in the patient's kitchen or sitting room, with the kitchen table as an operating table. A boiling pot was used as a sterilizer and pots and pans served as receptacles for instruments and supplies. Martin's doctor friends participated in these procedures as assistants, anesthetists, and nurses. In the late 1800s, this was how physicians learned to be surgeons: by declaring a willingness to perform urgent and emergent operations in cases where the diagnosis and treatment were obvious. At the time young physicians had minimal opportunities to learn through observing established surgeons. As a regrettable consequence, few physicians interested in surgery became skilled practitioners early in their careers. But because of his tenacity, Martin did become a very good surgeon.[7]

Dancing Lessons

It occurred to Martin that it might be an asset to him socially if he could learn to dance, so he enrolled at a local dancing academy. To his surprise, dancing was a vigorous activity and, combining the lessons with frequent long walks around Chicago, he became more fit. As discussed in earlier chapters, before coming to Chicago for medical school he had always been active, exercising strenuously outdoors at work and play. In his words, "...my health and spirits were best when I was engaged in some physical activity."[8] Throughout medical school and internship, he had led a relatively sedentary lifestyle, which left him restless and stale. Although he obviously enjoyed the challenge of being a physician, he often looked back with joy to the vigorous lifestyle he led in the first 20 years of his life.[8]

First Publications at Age 25

While working with Dr. D. R. Brower at St. Joseph's Hospital in Chicago, Martin published his first manuscripts. Under Dr. Brower's supervision, they were initiating a new treatment of nervous diseases, developed by Dr. S. Weir Mitchell, of Philadelphia, PA, called the "rest cure." In addition to prolonged rest, massage was part of the therapy. On researching the literature, Martin discovered minimal information was available about massage, so he decided to write a manuscript about the subject to enlighten the medical community. In addition to reviewing the available literature, he spoke in detail with a few Swedish masseurs and masseuses and produced an acceptable manuscript. This investigative approach is an example from early in his medical career of Martin's uncanny ability to identify a problem, research that problem, and outline a solution, something he first learned working on the farm and teaching school. He submitted the manuscript, titled "Massage—Its Application," to the *Chicago Medical Journal & Examiner,* and to his great pride it was accepted for publication. Dr. Brower was so impressed that he asked Martin to write a report about an interesting case of a brain tumor. This article, too, was accepted for publication in the same journal—"Case of Epileptiform Convulsion and Paralysis Due to Syphilitic Tumor of the Cortex in Motor Area," by Franklin H. Martin and D. R. Brower.[9]

Helps Form the Chicago South-Side Medico-Social Society

In the spring of 1883 another physician, Dr. Edmund J. Doering, came to Martin's office and suggested that they organize a medical club with an exclusive membership of young physicians from the south side of

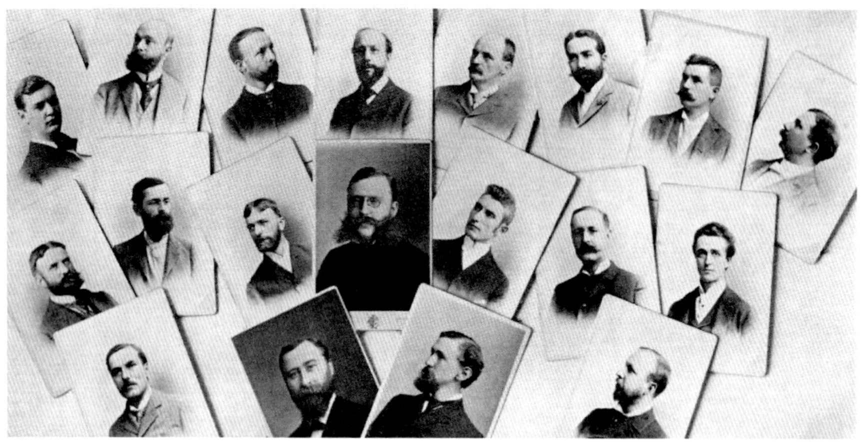

6.2 Chicago South-Side Medico-Social Society members. Martin is third from the right in the middle row. Lorenzo Potter is third from the left in the middle row. Edmund Doering, President of the Society, is fourth from the left in the middle row.

Chicago. Only doctors approved by the charter members would be eligible for membership. Martin was in favor of the club and only asked that Dr. Potter be included as a charter member. It was to be named The Chicago South-Side Medico-Social Society.

The introduction to the society's constitution read, "…on the second day of May 1883, for the promotion of good fellowship, harmony and union among its members; for the advancement of medical science, and for the maintenance of a high professional standard."[10] Initially, the organization had only eight members, and it was not until 10 years later that the membership reached 21 physicians (Figure 6.2). At every meeting, a member presented a scientific paper, and every member present was required to discuss the paper without prepared notes for at least five minutes. The group took the presentations and discussions seriously. Because most members were unaccustomed to speaking in public, this drill was of inestimable advantage to them when they spoke elsewhere.

Members laboriously prepared and presented draft manuscripts to the society. Papers deemed of appropriate quality were recommended to local organizations for presentation at their meetings. If accepted, other members of the society would be on hand for the discussion. Because of the level of preparation, the presentations routinely were successful.

Interestingly, according to Martin, for more than 30 years other societies were unaware of The Chicago South-Side Medico-Social Society members' intense preparation for their presentations. The society's well-prepared papers were held in high esteem, and, as a result, members were readily accepted for admission to other prestigious societies. Martin believed that their self-disciplined approach to preparing and giving presentations influenced medicine in their community.[10]

REFERENCES

1. Martin, F. H. (1933). *The Joy of Living: An Autobiography,* vol.1 (p. 218). New York, NY: Doubleday, Doran & Co.
2. Ibid., pp. 219-222.
3. Ibid., pp. 222-225.
4. Ibid., p. 228.
5. Ibid., p. 41.
6. Ibid., pp. 235-236.
7. Ibid., pp. 230-231.
8. Ibid., p. 234.
9. Ibid., p. 235.
10. Ibid., pp. 236-238.

Chapter 7

Courtship and Marriage to Isabelle Hollister

oon noised ~~about~~ those ~~...~~ thought
that the Corlins had brought
visitors on Sunday Every boo
claim on the big bend.
the raising on Saturday. Volunteers
~~hands~~ were busy from all the neig
the week, felling trees, hewing ~~the~~ addition
the shape for the new house. Early
of Saturday a dozen or more st
and boys were on hand to construc
house. ~~A~~ cellar had been dug in
~~f~~ ready to be encased with sto
logs had been sunk in be
reached a bed of solid clay beneath th
, lumber had been brought fro
mill and a fine lot of dry
been contributed by generous neighbors
~~...~~ ready to compete with s
that had been bro
sturdy oxen

neighbors.

From Indian boy common cons
of the game
for the day. No time was
sal ~~devotions~~ came - the great logs
about their necks a
iron chains of the faithful oxen

Isabelle's Background

Martin's marriage to Isabelle Hollister (Figure 7.1) had a profound effect on his life and career. Isabelle was the daughter of Dr. John H. Hollister, professor of pathology at the Chicago Medical College, where Martin had attended medical school. Isabelle was intelligent, learned, and Martin's intellectual equal. Martin believed that he would never be affluent, that he was without a social or financial position or influence, and that he had no cultural background, no personal charm, and no family prestige.[1] Isabelle and her parents embodied those characteristics, and she brought those attributes to their marriage. She insisted that Martin lead a balanced life and that their evenings be reserved for enjoying the arts and pursuits outside of medicine. He said of her influence on him, "It was the 'Education of the Wisconsin Boy' under a most discriminating tutor."[2]

Courtship and Marriage

Martin first noticed Isabelle when he saw her perform in an amateur play at a private club in a small hall on the south side of Chicago and decided he should make her acquaintance. Isabelle played the part of a parlor maid, and in Martin's eyes she was sensational. Soon thereafter, at a reception at a local club, they were formally introduced. They danced and afterward became involved in a long conversation. He felt she was an engaging conversationalist; he admired her ability to hold down her end of any discussion, regardless of the topic, although at this time she was only 18 and he was 26. Regrettably, Isabelle and her parents were leaving the following day on a long vacation out west to Yellowstone Park, leaving him without a way to continue their relationship. It was Martin's assessment that he fell in love with Isabelle almost immediately, and he spent the next two years courting her.[3]

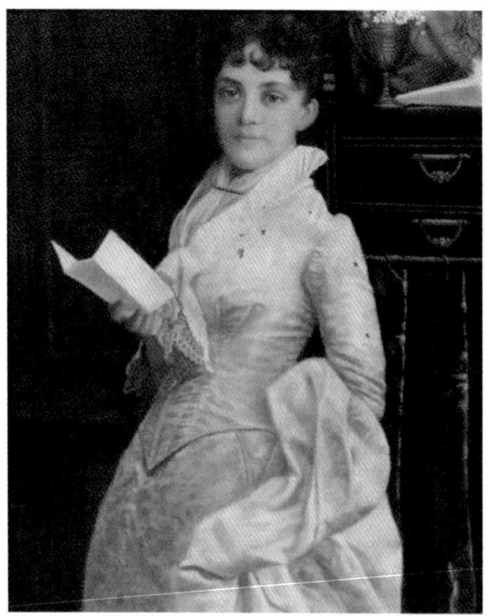
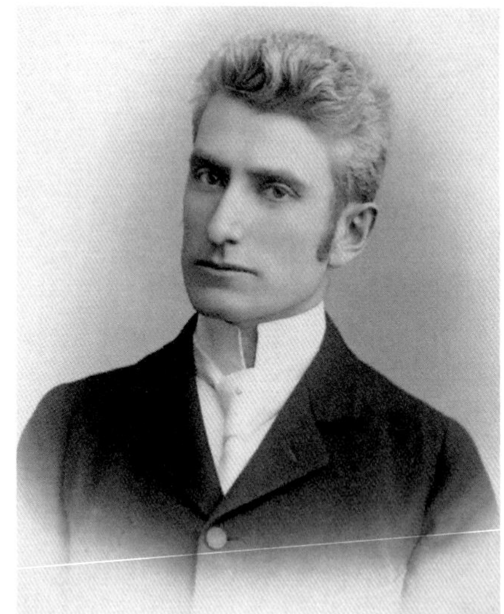

7.1. Isabelle Hollister Martin (left) and Franklin Martin (right) at about the time of their marriage.

Upon Isabelle's return, she invited Martin to her home to spend an evening with some friends. With this invitation, Martin became a changed man, and his friends at the Lords' boardinghouse believed he was in a perpetual state of ecstasy. A few of the observant women even suggested he was in love, which was, in fact, true. Martin enjoyed the evening at the Hollisters' home, but there was no opportunity for the couple to have a private conversation. Over the next few months, they had occasional interactions that he characterized more as sparring matches than conventional conversations. He was falling hopelessly in love but did not have the courage to make his feelings known. He began spending more time with Isabelle and believed she was beginning to welcome his companionship. "She was an intellectual treat to my starving soul! Her merry wit...her enjoyment of life...and her appreciation of the best of everything, filled me with a new joy. The realization of her worth was making me a better, a stronger, and a different man."[4] He felt at a distinct disadvantage discussing music and books with Isabelle because of his ignorance of such topics. He later suspected that she was subtly beginning the task of educating him in the liberal arts. After an enjoyable day with their friends at a baseball game, followed by a party and fireworks, he proposed marriage. But she believed they needed further time for reflection and refused to say yes.[4]

Despite her rebuff, his courtship continued unabated, and Martin felt encouraged enough to approach her father about his desire to marry his daughter. Regrettably, he had not consulted with Isabelle before talking with Dr. Hollister and was chastised for this behavior the next time they talked.[5] As a result of this conversation, Isabelle's parents decided she should visit her friends on the East Coast, during which time there would be no communications between Isabelle and Franklin. If, after returning to Chicago, she wished to reinstate the relationship, they would support her decision.

On her return to Chicago, initially Isabelle did not contact Martin, but after a chance meeting while walking with a friend on Michigan Avenue, he requested a rendezvous to have a serious talk. At that time, Isabelle confessed her feelings for Martin and her desire to proceed with marriage plans. During a meeting between Isabelle, her parents, and Martin it was decided that the couple should wait a year before making a final decision. If at the end of a year they still wished to marry, the couple would have her parents' support.[6] As Martin describes the next few months, the couple grew closer. Their mutual appreciation of the arts and their enjoyment of philosophical discussions fortified their bond.[7] The Hollisters ultimately capitulated and wholeheartedly supported the union. The couple was wed May 27, 1886. Martin was rattled by the proceedings and was unable to complete his vows. The minister ignored his blunder and proceeded with the ritual. After the ceremony they retired to their new home at 3308 Rhodes Avenue, near the Hollisters.[8] Interestingly, none of Martin's family from Wisconsin was on the guest list.

ISABELLE'S TALENTS

Isabelle brought many interesting and useful talents to their relationship. For instance, in Martin's research on uterine fibroids, he needed a text translated from French into English, which Isabelle was able to do easily. Also, Martin was having significant problems managing their money, and on confessing this difficulty to Isabelle, she immediately took over the family finances. Her assessment was that he was a spendthrift with no understanding of the value of money. For example, Martin thought he had no more than $50 in debts when, in fact, he owed $1,000. Under Isabelle's guidance they were able to pay off his debt and learn to live within their means. Working together on improving their financial circumstances also improved their sense of solidarity.[9]

Because of the impact of the new and important field of bacteriology on the practice of medicine, Martin had decided to take a course in bacteriology and, much to his surprise, Isabelle announced that she would like to take the course with him. Every morning for weeks they listened to lectures and learned about the function of a bacteriology laboratory. It was obviously an interesting experience for both, and one that had a positive impact on their relationship.[10]

Marriage: Its Positive Effect on Martin's Health

Martin's relationship with Isabelle had a profound effect on both his professional and personal life. By his assessment, without her he would never have accomplished all he was able to in his lifetime. She was his touchstone, the person to whom he turned when he needed to make difficult decisions and needed support.

For the first few years of their marriage, Isabelle allowed Martin to manage his career and life as he saw fit. But after four years of marriage, when Isabelle noticed his unfit and anemic appearance, she took matters into her own hands. Martin was not in favor of vacations, and he and Isabelle participated in few leisure activities. One day, as a diversion, she took Martin out to lunch and to a Cubs' baseball game, which they both enjoyed so much that they returned for games every three weeks if the team was playing in Chicago. Martin said of the experience, "…an intangible something brought health, extreme joy of living, and 'pep' that I had not enjoyed since my labors in the brickyard or on the farm."[11]

In 1898, Martin became a charter member of the Midlothian Country Club south of Chicago, and he and Isabelle became avid golfers (Figure 7.2). For 15 years, during the summer they stayed in the living quarters of the clubhouse along with many other members. Martin was enthusiastic about golf as a sport because he believed it gave ambitious men and women the opportunity to enjoy some exercise in the open air, something he thoroughly enjoyed his entire life.[12]

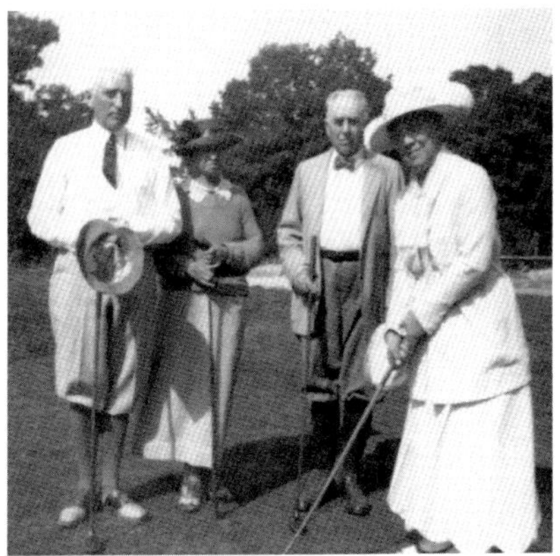
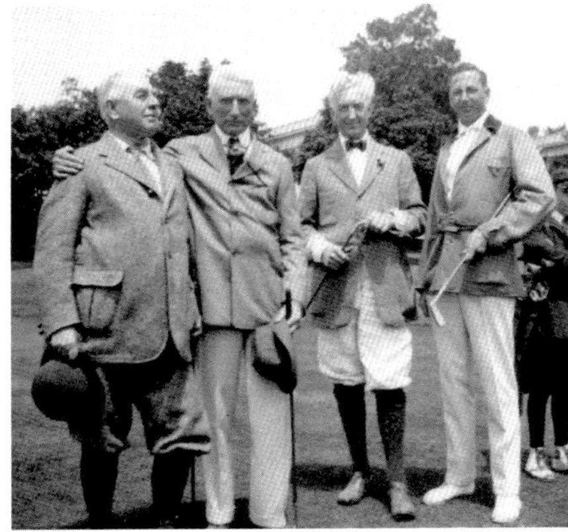

7.2. Martin golfing with friends. In the first photograph (a) he is on the left-hand side and Isabelle is preparing to hit the ball. In (b) he is second from the left.

Isabelle, the Vacation Planner

After six years of marriage with no vacations, in 1892 Isabelle and Martin planned a riverboat trip from New Orleans to St. Louis as a belated honeymoon. Considering Martin's dislike of being away from work, there is little doubt that Isabelle made the arrangements. The trip was a complete success, and the Martins both enjoyed it thoroughly.[13]

In 1894, after 10 years of working 16-hour days, Martin found himself exhausted, with a lack of keenness for work or adventure. "I found myself becoming irritable and irascible in my contacts with some of my associates."[14] Isabelle, sensing his need for a break, suggested a summer trip to Alaska with stops along the West Coast of the U.S., where Martin attended the annual meeting of the American Medical Association (AMA) in San Francisco. At this meeting Martin was, to his surprise, elected to the chairmanship of the section of the AMA on obstetrics and the diseases of women—a prestigious appointment for a young man of 37.

Following the AMA meeting, the Martins took a steamer excursion through the fjords of Alaska, which Martin described as a restful and stimulating two weeks. They returned to Chicago on the Canadian Pacific Railroad through the Canadian Rockies. The trip changed Martin's mental attitude. He realized that his troubles were of little consequence, and that "The perspective of things worth while obscured the small, irritating problems."[14] He believed he was a new man and ready for the abundant work that awaited him. This enlarged perspective served him well the remainder of his life. He never missed the opportunity to travel and reap its benefits, especially when he was able to combine business with pleasure.[14]

The following year, Martin was invited to the British Medical Association meeting in London, England. He and Isabelle expanded the 10-day meeting into five weeks, touring France and Great Britain. He and Isabelle—one suspects mostly Isabelle—laboriously worked out an itinerary for the entire trip. Neither of them had ever been to Europe, and they therefore included the usual sites on their program. Martin said of the trip, "It was of course the greatest adventure we have ever had."[15] A style of travel was established that he and Isabelle would repeat on numerous occasions throughout their lifetime together. Besides its other benefits, traveling and seeking new adventures together was a bonding experience for the couple.[15]

Isabelle's Impact on Franklin

In 1897 Martin looked back over the first 11 years of his marriage to Isabelle and "...realized that in recent years I had been under the sympathetic guidance of a brilliant, intellectual, and highly educated woman, whom I had taken 'for better or worse' eleven short years before."[16] In his words, "With her blessed influence, she had established a rule that 'after six o'clock at night all talk of shop must stop,' and that our spare time should be devoted to reading good literature, hearing good music, and associating with people of serious character and with a cultural tendency."[16] In his mind, this ritual helped compensate for his lack of an earlier liberal arts education. It was not always possible to eliminate all shop talk at 6:00 pm because they often entertained medical students as dinner guests. The students and their friends were always welcome at the Martin household.[16]

Dr. C. Jeff Miller, a friend of the couple, said of the Martins' relationship, "...how necessary she was to his happiness, and how much his success has been due to her sound judgment, loyalty, and companionship."[17]

Even before they were married, Isabelle began exposing Franklin to classical music. For their entire life together, they attended Chicago Symphony Orchestra concerts and the opera. Before meeting Isabelle,

Martin had never attended such events, but he rapidly became infatuated with them.

Throughout their marriage, on many evenings the couple read magazine articles and books aloud to each other, including Guizot's *History of Civilization in Europe, Causes of the Civil War in America,* Washington Irving's *Life of George Washington,* and *The Life and Letters of Charles Darwin.* In his words, "The leisure of those hours, the changing trend of thought, and the knowledge gained compelled us to a broader vision, and to great enjoyment of life."[16] This activity helped deepen the bond between the two. Of their relationship Dr. George W. Crile later said, "Franklin Martin did not fight and work and dream alone, as Isabelle Hollister Martin has advised, moderated, and conciliated this colorful personality."[18]

ISABELLE'S SUPPORT OF MAJOR PROJECTS

In 1905, when Martin was in the initial stages of developing a new surgical journal, *Surgery, Gynecology & Obstetrics,* he told Isabelle of his "new dream." Initially she was opposed to the project because in her opinion he already was working beyond a reasonable capacity. He argued "that the plan was mine, that I would be annoyed if someone else were assigned to carry it out, and, anyway, it would always be on my mind. It would be better to assume the burden myself than to fret because of the failure of someone else."[19] Isabelle was upset to the point of tears with this new endeavor, but Martin's enthusiasm eventually won her over to his side.[19]

Five years later, in 1910, Martin conceived of a Clinical Congress of Surgeons of North America. When he laid out his plan before Isabelle, she gave her full support and encouragement. She did say, however, that she worried that her sympathy for the project would doom it to failure.[20]

LATER IN LIFE

Isabelle and Franklin remained close companions for the remainder of his life. In the last five years of Martin's life, they made frequent trips to visit his family in Wisconsin, often bringing along friends from Chicago. Martin seemed to want to show both Isabelle and their friends where he had spent the first 20 years of his life and demonstrate why those years brought him great joy. These trips will be discussed in greater detail in Chapter 15.

In the last paragraph of his autobiography, Martin again praised his wife, saying that he had enjoyed "the blessed companionship of a wonderful woman—Isabelle."[21]

REFERENCES

1. Martin, F. H. (1933). *The Joy of Living: An Autobiography,* vol. 1 (p. 240). New York, NY: Doubleday, Doran & Co.
2. Ibid., p. 364.
3. Ibid., pp. 238-240.
4. Ibid., pp. 241-248.
5. Ibid., pp. 264-266.
6. Ibid., pp. 275-278.
7. Ibid., p. 281.
8. Ibid., pp. 284-286.
9. Ibid., pp. 286-288.
10. Ibid., p. 312.
11. Ibid., p. 318.
12. Ibid., pp. 371-373.
13. Ibid., pp. 323-324.
14. Ibid., pp. 335-343.
15. Ibid., pp. 346-347 and pp. 352-353.
16. Ibid., pp. 361-364.
17. Miller. C. J. (1935). Franklin H. Martin—the friend. *Bull Am Coll Surg*, 20(2), 45.
18. Crile, G. W. Foreword. In Martin, F.H. (1933). *The Joy of Living: An Autobiography,* vol. 1 (p. xiv). New York, NY: Doubleday, Doran & Co.
19. Martin, F. H. (1933). *The Joy of Living: An Autobiography,* vol. 1 (p. 398). New York, NY: Doubleday, Doran & Co.
20. Ibid., p. 403.
21. Martin, F. H. (1933). *The Joy of Living: An Autobiography,* vol. 2 (p. 468). New York, NY: Doubleday, Doran & Co.

Chapter 8

Exploring New Medical Therapies and Learning to Operate

oon noised ab
that the Corbins those brought
Iiestons on Sunday had Every boo
claim on the big bend. Volunteer
the raising on Saturday.
~~hands~~ were busy from all the neig
the week, felling trees, hewing ~~the~~ addition
the shape for the new house. Early
ig of Saturday a dozen or more sti
and boys were on hand to construct
house. A cellar had been dug in th
~~fou~~ ready to be encased with ston
cabin logs had been sunk in hem
reached a bed of solid clay beneath the
il, lumber had been brought from
our mill and a fine lot of dry
been contributed by generous neighbors
ver ~~[illegible]~~ ready to compete with Se
Sunday oxen that had been brou
neighbors.
Iron Mother by common consent
foreman for the day. No time was
all directions came the great logs of the year
iron chains about their necks a
of the faithful oxen

IMPACT OF LAWSON TAIT ON DECISION TO PERFORM OPERATIONS

Because of his work in the Department of Gynecology and the Diseases of Women at the South Side Dispensary, Martin became interested in performing the operations that his patients required. Although he frequently performed minor procedures, at the time he had never performed a major abdominal operation; but he was prepared to do so if an appropriate patient was identified.

Late in 1883, he saw a patient with severe abdominal pain from an ovarian mass and recommended to her that she have an oophorectomy. Because of the severity of her pain, she readily agreed. He reviewed the available literature about the work of British surgeon Dr. Lawson Tait, whose patients had a significantly lower incidence of postoperative infections and excellent results following abdominal operations. Dr. Tait was ruthless in his opposition to Sir Joseph Lister's theory of antiseptic surgery and his use of carbolic acid spray in the operating room to decrease surgical infection rates. Instead, Tait advocated for aseptic surgery, and although he did not reveal all the underlying features of his operative protocols, we do know that he adhered to high standards of cleanliness in his operating room. He sterilized his instruments and suture material by boiling them in water and scrubbed the skin with soap and water before making the incision. Only his hands were allowed in the operative field. In addition, "He was extremely skilled and dexterous; his incisions were short, just large enough to permit him to do his work...no assistants touched the field of operation."[1] Using this protocol, his patient survival rate equaled Sir Lister's.

Martin described the underlying principle of Tait's approach, that "everything that came in direct contact with the wound must be absolutely germ free."[1] We now know, of course, that such techniques do not keep the wound free of bacteria, but they do keep the concentration of bacteria low enough that infections occur infrequently, which partially explains why both techniques had positive effects on post-operative infection rates.

Martin continued to follow the bacteriological literature about hand cleanliness as he prepared for his first abdominal operation. It had been revealed that even after immersing hands in a strong antiseptic, an abundance of bacteria remained in hand scrapings and beneath the nails. Only after scrubbing the hands and nails with an antiseptic followed by rinsing could the bacteria levels be reduced significantly. In view of this data, Martin scrubbed and rinsed his hands before operations. He used a modification of Lister's protocols to prepare the operating room and during the operation. In addition, he used a surgical protocol that was a modification of Tait's operative procedure. One of Martin's close friends, Dr. Frederic A. Besley, observed that at this time Martin was one of the first surgeons to use antiseptic and later aseptic technique in the operating room.[2] The thoroughness with which he studied the work of other surgeons and bacteriologists before performing this operation was unusual at this time.

The procedure was performed in a large room of an apartment near his office. The patient tolerated the operation, a bilateral oophorectomy, without complications, but regrettably died of sepsis on the second postoperative day. Martin was despondent. Although he had done everything known at that time to avoid infection, he had performed the operation in isolation without the advantage of advice and assistance from more experienced surgeons.[1]

Although he continued to perform minor procedures, it wasn't until two years later, in 1885, that Martin performed his second abdominal operation. At the time of the operation, the patient was found to have a large ovarian mass that on aspiration was revealed to be infected. The mass was sutured to the peritoneum at the site of the abdominal incision and a plug of gauze placed in the original incision down to the level of the mass. The operation was then terminated. Three days later, in a second procedure, the gauze plug was removed, the mass identified where it was adhered to the abdominal wall, and an incision was made to drain the pus. A third operation was required to drain residual pus, after which the patient made an uneventful recovery.[3]

Here is another clear example of Martin's ability to make a diagnosis, then do a thorough search of the literature on the topic and perform the indicated procedure using appropriate precautions. Few physicians at this juncture in American medicine would have been capable of planning and performing an abdominal operation under these circumstances without the benefit of consulting more experienced surgeons, most of whom lived great distances away and were not easily contacted.

Use of Electricity in the Treatment of Uterine Fibroids

Not all the unique medical treatments that Martin evaluated resulted in an effective new therapy. In 1884 he became aware of the work of the Frenchman Prof. George Apostoli on the use of galvanic current (continuous, unidirectional electricity) in the treatment of uterine fibroids. It was Professor Apostoli's large text on the treatment of uterine fibroids with galvanic electricity that Isabelle had translated from French to English for Martin. Martin investigated the field of electricity and the theory of its use in the treatment of uterine fibroids, especially when there was symptomatic hemorrhage. Professor Apostoli answered all of Martin's written inquiries in detail. For more than a year, Martin worked on the design and construction of the apparatus necessary to treat uterine fibroids with electricity. Once he was satisfied with the safety of the instrumentation, he decided to begin using it on patients. He considered the outcome for his first three patients to be successful, which he reported in the *Journal of the American Medical Association*.[4]

Over time, Martin modified the apparatus to include improved intrauterine electrodes, but, in the end, he abandoned the therapy because of the results of an experiment he conducted in 1891 on hens' eggs. Although not exceedingly well designed because he did not include a group with no electricity, the experiment gave him the information he felt he needed: he found that when fertile eggs were treated with galvanic electrical current, like that used to treat uterine fibroid patients, such treatment was uniformly fatal to the chicken embryos. Seventy percent of the eggs treated with faradic electricity (alternating current) produced live chicks. He assumed that galvanic electricity would have a similar effect on a human ovum and therefore stopped using it to treat uterine fibroids.[5]

Expansion of His Clinical Practice

By the start of 1885, Martin's practice had substantially increased in size, which he attributed to his patients referring friends to his care. He continued to perform minor operations on his clinic patients.

With the expansion of his patient base, he began seeing patients with perplexing problems that required him to review the medical literature in detail. He believed that a thorough review of specific medical topics was a crucial aspect of a physician's practice, and that it must be done honestly and thoroughly to avoid misleading conclusions. Martin said, "...conducting actual research in literature...has since been of inestimable value to me, for it has made me realize the importance and intricacy of such work, the worthlessness of inaccurate research, and the value of an honest, comprehensive job."[6] Such thorough research made it feasible for him to initiate new therapies without consulting directly with known experts in a specific medical field—as he had done in his approach to learning aseptic surgery.

Hystero-Neurasthenia

By 1887, Martin had spent years treating women with a symptom complex where, in his words, "Many of the women had lost courage, they were partially bedridden, their strength was depleted, and their initiative was practically at the lowest ebb."[7] He gave this complex of symptoms the name hystero-neurasthenia, or nervous exhaustion of women, because he believed the symptoms were the result of "a partial or general nervous inefficiency, or perversion, of the nerves controlling the organs peculiar to women."[7] His recommended therapy was the rest cure developed by Dr. S. Weir Mitchell of Philadelphia for the treatment of general neurasthenia. The therapy involved rest, an appropriate diet, seclusion, and sleep. To this regimen Martin added electrical current therapy and massage. This occurred before his decision to abandon electrical current therapy. Many of his patients improved with the outlined therapy.[7] Because of his misdiagnosis of the etiology of the syndrome, the term hystero-neurasthenia was never well accepted and fell into disuse. In many ways, in this case he was not following his own advice of thoroughly researching the literature to avoid making misleading conclusions.

Intellectual Approach to Patient Care

By 1888, after seven years of medical practice, a few areas were of particular concern to Martin. His medical practice, with its increasing number of patients requiring operative therapy, was of paramount importance, as was the management of the essential functions of his office. Another important aspect of his practice was preparing manuscripts based on his clinical work for publication in medical journals, which involved extensive research of the available literature and long hours of writing.

His patients and their individual problems were his main concern and intensely interested him. He enjoyed meeting patients, reviewing their symptoms, and studying their ailments. He also cared about their fears and anxieties. The same deep-seated concern engaged him every time he prepared for and performed an operation.

Martin's level of absorption in the function of his practice, in his patients, and in his writings factored significantly in his successful career. Everywhere you look in his life story, there is the same level of intensity and intellectual involvement.[8]

An example of how others viewed Martin's abilities is Dr. William Mayo's reminiscence of visiting Martin's clinic: "I remember well the morning that I first had the privilege of seeing Dr. Martin perform some most delicate operations with skill and precision. I was greatly impressed, and from that time I was an attendant at his clinics whenever the opportunity arose."[9]

REFERENCES

1. Martin, F. H. (1933). *The Joy of Living: An Autobiography,* vol. 1 (pp. 248-255). New York, NY: Doubleday, Doran & Co.
2. Besley, F. A. (1935). Franklin H. Martin—the surgeon. *Bull Am Coll Surg,* 20(2), 41.
3. Martin, F. H. (1933). *The Joy of Living: An Autobiography,* vol. 1 (pp. 278-280). New York, NY: Doubleday, Doran & Co.
4. Ibid., pp. 257-260, 274-275, 283, and 288.
5. Ibid., pp. 321-322.
6. Ibid., pp. 273-275.
7. Ibid., pp. 291-296.
8. Ibid., pp. 301-302.
9. Mayo, W. J. Foreword. In: Martin, F. H. (1933). *The Joy of Living: An Autobiography,* vol. 1 (pp. xi-xii). New York, NY: Doubleday, Doran & Co.

Chapter 9

Mid-Career Highlights

oon noised a[bout]
that the Corbins those ~~[struck]~~ brought t
Irishins on Sunday had. Every boa
claim on the big bend.
the raising on Saturday. Volunteers
~~hands~~ were busy from all the neig[h]
and addition ~~the~~
the week, felling trees, hewing. Early
ir shape for the new house.
g of Saturday a dozen or more sli
nd boys were on hand to construc[t]
ouse. A cellar had been dug in th
~~for~~ is ready to be encased with sto[ne]
alin logs had been sunk in ben[?]
eached a bed of solid clay beneath th
il, lumber had been brought from
aw mill and a fine lot of dry o[ak]
been contributed by generous neighbors
er ~~oxen~~ ready to compete with Su[nday]
that had been brou[ght]
Sunday oxen
neighbors.
Ira Irishm by common cons[ent]
of the gang
foreman for the day. No time was
all directions came the great logs
iron chains about their necks a
of the faithful oxen
cheerf

American Medical Association Presentation and "Ruthless" Reply to Criticism

As a member of the Chicago Medical Society, the Chicago Gynecological Society, the Chicago South Side Medico-Social Society, the American Medical Association (AMA), and the American Gynecological Society, Martin often gave presentations based on his clinical work. In addition, he took a keen interest in others' contributions. It was his habit to review any available abstracts before a meeting so that he could more effectively critique the podium presentations. But such critiques did not always meet with a positive response. In his words: "Impelled by my youthful enthusiasm to criticize honestly, I fear I did not realize at the time the ruthlessness of my manner, nor the fact that I was jeopardizing friendships of long standing."[1] Dr. Edmund J. Doering, President of the Chicago South Side Medico-Social Society, admonished: "Martin, why are you so hard on these friends of ours? Now you must apologize to that man!"[1] Although he accepted Dr. Doering's advice as well intended, Martin sometimes resented what he interpreted as interference. In most instances, Martin eventually would apologize and decide to become more tactful. But regrettably, when faced again with what he interpreted as a poor-quality presentation, he still was likely to make undiplomatic comments.

At the annual meeting of the AMA in 1890, Martin presented a paper titled "A Plea for Early Vaginal Hysterectomy for Cancer of the Uterus." The paper was based on his clinical experience and included a review of the literature. The audience responded favorably, but Dr. Thaddeus Reamy, a well-known and respected senior gynecologist, discussed Martin's paper in very uncomplimentary terms. In Martin's view, Dr. Reamy presented no concrete criticisms, but rather unleashed a tirade of personal epithets. Dr. Reamy looked to the audience for support and received none. Obviously, the association's members were unhappy with his tirade. The same man had, in the past, been similarly critical of presentations, in particular those given by young authors.

Martin began his rebuttal by stating that he hoped that in the future his mind would be open to progress, unlike his antagonist, whose mind was closed to the work and efforts of young surgeons. He said that he hoped in the future scientific papers would be discussed on their merit alone and not on the prejudices of the discussant. Martin ended by criticizing Dr. Reamy for denouncing Martin only for his youthfulness and not for the quality of his work.

Martin later realized that it would have been more dignified to ignore Dr. Reamy's insulting remarks, but he "lacked that wisdom." Instead, he was "ruthless and indiscreet" in his response. Dr. Reamy then charged the podium, railing accusations. At this point Dr. Nathan S. Davis, founder of the AMA, requested that both men accompany him on a walk. Dr. Davis soundly criticized Martin for insulting "the white hairs of age," and criticized Reamy for his uncomplimentary personal remarks about Martin. In the end, Martin and Reamy shook hands and became friends.[1]

Regrettably, this was not the first, nor would it be the last, time that Martin would be indiscreet or tactless when discussing presentations or making comments at national meetings or conferences. Interestingly, his outbursts did not always have a negative impact. His strong and sometimes controversial statements in support of the American College of Surgeons (ACS) in response to challenges by the AMA and other institutions were a major factor in the College becoming a dominant force in American medicine. There is little doubt that without his sturdy, unrelenting support of ACS policies, the AMA ultimately would have become the spokesman for American surgery.

Improving Operative Therapy

It was Martin's assessment in 1892 that hysterectomy was the most appropriate therapy for the severe symptoms of pain and hemorrhage experienced by some patients with fibroid tumors of the uterus, despite the high mortality rate for that procedure compared with other abdominal operations. It was Martin's opinion that intra-abdominal hemorrhage following inadequate ligation of the uterine vessels during abdominal hysterectomy was the main reason for the increased mortality rate. Another surgeon suggested a solution, which was to incise the broad ligament and identify the uterine vessels directly, apply a clamp to the vessels, and ligate the individual vessels. This change in procedure decreased the mortality rate from 40 percent to less than 5 percent, and eventually to between 2 and 3 percent, commensurate with other abdominal operations. Later in his surgical career, Martin performed a series of 100 hysterectomies without a mortality.[2]

Also, in 1892 Martin decided that simple ligation of the uterine arteries, without hysterectomy, would markedly decrease the blood supply to the uterus and decrease uterine bleeding in patients with severe bleeding. In the next two years he successfully performed this operation in six patients. The procedure was in use for a brief period but as major abdominal surgery, such as hysterectomy, became safer, simple ligation of the uterine arteries fell into disuse.[2]

Martin's receptiveness to learning new procedures and modifications of existing operations served him well throughout his career. He was a leader in the development of abdominal surgery, particularly gynecologic abdominal surgery, despite his lack of interaction with other, more experienced abdominal surgeons. He compensated for that deficit by staying up to date with the medical literature and regularly attending regional and national meetings. Dr. Frederic A. Besley described Martin's surgical technique as: "meticulous, his handling of tissues gentle and dexterous; though a fearless and rapid operator, he was never over radical, and his conclusions relative to pathological conditions and their operability were based on sound surgical judgment."[3]

Becoming Famous in 1895: Invitation to the British Medical Association Annual Meeting

While attending the annual meeting of the British Medical Association in London, England, Martin was invited to participate in the annual dinner of the British Gynecological Society. On arrival at the dinner, he was greeted by a friend, Prof. August Martin of Berlin, Germany, who was the guest of honor. Martin had met Professor Martin eight years earlier at the International Medical Congress in Washington, DC. The professor had arranged for Martin to sit with him at the head table, along with Dr. Lawson Tait, Sir Joseph Lister, and other distinguished physicians. Martin was introduced and a long list of his accomplishments noted. Although the audience encouraged him to speak, at that time he declined.

When Sir Lister was introduced, the audience gave him a standing ovation; Lister responded with brief remarks. Meanwhile, Dr. Tait muttered some disparaging remarks about Lister. As mentioned earlier, Tait was an unyielding critic of Lister, asserting that the only significant effect of spraying carbolic acid as an antiseptic was to prevent contamination of the wound with airborne bacteria. Tait believed that wound decontamination could be better achieved by washing and scrubbing the skin and surgeons' hands with soap and water and sterilizing the instruments in boiling water. Tait maintained that he alone was responsible for establishing this principle.

Martin thought Tait was unfair in giving Lister insufficient credit for being the first physician to describe an effective technique for decreasing bacterial contamination. This unfair behavior had irritated Martin for some time. When the hosts again asked Martin to speak, he came forward. He praised both Lister and Tait for their techniques but gave Lister credit for first establishing the principle of excluding bacteria from surgical wounds as a means to control infection. He suggested that Tait should be a follower of Lister, not a critic. Echoing the host's toast to Lister, Martin toasted Tait, and the audience responded with approval. Tait came to the podium and made complimentary remarks about Martin's speech, and invited Martin to visit his clinic. Martin later regretted that prior commitments prevented him from accepting the offer.[4]

Martin's Review of the Improvements in Medical Care at the Turn of the Century

In a retrospective examination of the state of medicine in 1900, Martin reviewed some of the major advances in medical care that had occurred since the 1880s. He also looked back at his personal accomplishments during his first 20 years of practice. At 42 years old, his professional accomplishments, his family life, his physical activities, and his social connections all gave him great satisfaction. He believed his contributions to the medical literature and his teaching had been well received. But in view of the significant advances that were changing the practice of medicine and surgery from an art to a science, Martin still was dissatisfied with his personal accomplishments. Scientific studies had demonstrated the importance of careful diagnosis and the value of

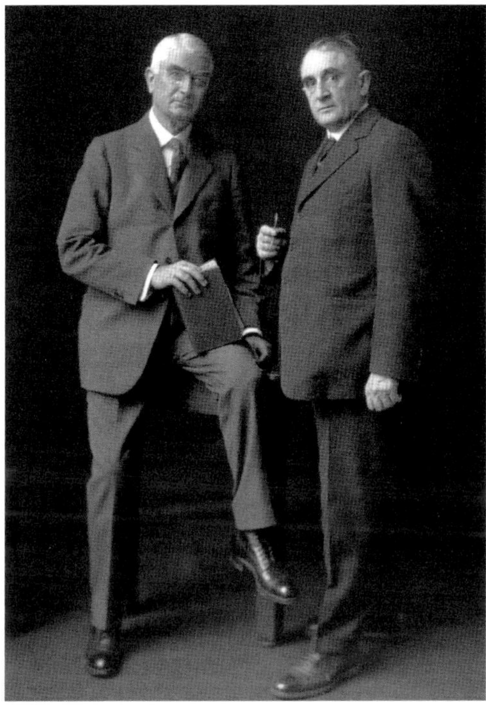

9.1. Drs. William J. (left) and Charles H. (right) Mayo.

preventative medicine. He was encouraged by the fact that physical therapy, fresh air, and exercise were becoming an important part of medical care. His review of the state of medicine in 1900 was well conceived and displayed an acute understanding of the topic.

In his memoir, Martin documented the improvement in the care of patients with tuberculosis, diphtheria, typhoid fever, and other infectious diseases, demonstrating his thorough knowledge of those conditions. His discussion of the 1895 discovery of X rays resulting in the establishment of radiology as a medical specialty, the demonstration of the pathology of perforating appendicitis, and the impact of the use of antisepsis in the operating room were all to the point. In summary he said, "How wonderful to have lived at this time, to have witnessed the ringing down of the curtain of a century of progress and to have touched the button that rang up the curtain of a new century of prospects!"[5]

Although Martin had not been involved in any of the most significant advances in medicine, he had done his part to improve the care of patients in the operating room, and he is to be praised for that. It is curious that in the list of accomplishments that gave him greatest satisfaction he included his strenuous physical activities—clearly a reference to his time as a farm laborer and brickmaker in rural Wisconsin. Except for his habit of going for long walks daily and playing golf, he certainly had not been involved in significant physical activities since leaving Wisconsin to begin his medical career.

The Mayo Brothers

Around 1902, Martin first visited the Mayo Clinic in Rochester, MN. He had heard enthusiastic reports about the Clinic and the Mayo brothers from many leading surgeons. At their initial meeting, Dr. Charles Mayo informed Martin that, without Martin's knowledge, he and his brother (Figure 9.1) had visited Martin's clinic at the Woman's Hospital in Chicago. Martin was impressed that they had done him this honor. He had dinner that evening at Charles Mayo's home and began a friendship with the Mayo brothers that continued for the rest of his life. Interestingly, their friendship began before he became famous for founding *Surgery, Gynecology & Obstetrics*, the Clinical Congress of Surgeons of North America, and the ACS. It is important to our understanding of Dr. Martin's place in the history of surgery in the U.S.—and, for that matter, the world—to remember that he was well-known and respected before 1905, when he embarked on those three major accomplishments. If the Mayo brothers visited his clinic before he visited theirs, that was clear evidence that he was having a significant impact on the practice of surgery in America before 1905.[6]

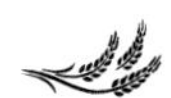

References

1. Martin, F. H. (1933). *The Joy of Living: An Autobiography,* vol. 1 (pp. 314-318). New York, NY: Doubleday, Doran & Co.
2. Ibid., pp. 327-330 and 381.
3. Besley, F. A. (1935). Franklin H. Martin—the surgeon. *Bull Am Coll Surg,* 20(2), 42.
4. Martin, F. H. (1933). *The Joy of Living: An Autobiography,* vol. 1 (pp. 347-352). New York, NY: Doubleday, Doran & Co.
5. Ibid., pp. 378-385.
6. Ibid., pp. 392-396.

Chapter 10

Other Significant Accomplishments

oon noised ab those ~~who~~ thought t
that the Corbins Sunday had Every boo
business on the big land.
claim on Saturday. Volunteers
the raising on all the neig
~~hands~~ were busy from addition
the week, felling trees, hewing and ~~the~~ Early
the shape for the new house.
g of Saturday a dozen or more sti
and boys were on hand to construc
house. A cellar had been dug in th
~~fo~~ is ready to be encased with ston
line logs had been sunk six fee
ached a bed of solid clay beneath th
il, lumber had been brought from
aw mill and a fine lot of dry o
been contributed by generous neighbors
en ~~oxen~~ ready to complete with Su
that had been brou
Sunday oxen
neighbors.
In mother's common cons
of the guns
woman for the day. No time was
all devotions came the great logs
iron chains about their necks a
of the faithful oxen
cheery

Founding of the Post-graduate Medical School and Hospital of Chicago

In 1888, at age 31, Martin was teaching postgraduate classes at the Chicago Policlinic. He enjoyed the experience tremendously. But he and a friend, Dr. W. Franklin Coleman, were dissatisfied with the clinic's administration, who they thought lacked the vision to develop a "much-needed" postgraduate medical school in Chicago. Their suggestions for improving the clinic were unfavorably received at faculty meetings.

After realizing how thoroughly dissatisfied they both were and how hopeless the situation was, Martin proposed that they organize a postgraduate school of medicine for Chicago. The two men surveyed other policlinic physicians and discovered that many members of the faculty also were dissatisfied and were waiting for someone to take the initiative. As was Martin's style, within a week he and Dr. Coleman had agreements from a tentative faculty of prominent, well-established Chicago physicians, allowing them to proceed. Dr. Frederic A. Besley maintained it was Martin's hope that the school would satisfy, among other objectives, "the need for disseminating the rapidly increasing knowledge of aseptic surgery."[1]

The preliminary organizational meeting occurred September 12, 1888. A board of directors was named, with Dr. Coleman as secretary and Martin as treasurer. Three months later the group rented a four-story building in downtown Chicago. At the same time the school leaders arranged to publish an official school journal, *The North American Practitioner*, which they envisioned as a highly scientific journal for the Middle West of the U.S. The school opened as planned April 1, 1889.[2]

Martin and Dr. Coleman identified the need for a graduate medical school and opened the facility in less than eight months. This was an amazing accomplishment for a 31-year-old physician who had only

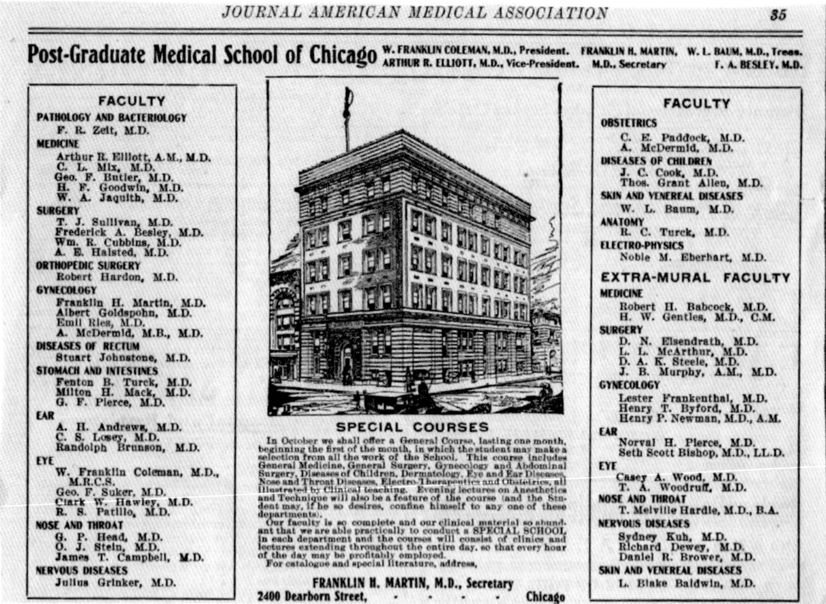

JOURNAL AMERICAN MEDICAL ASSOCIATION 35

Post-Graduate Medical School of Chicago

W. FRANKLIN COLEMAN, M.D., President. ARTHUR R. ELLIOTT, M.D., Vice-President. FRANKLIN H. MARTIN, M.D., Secretary. W. L. BAUM, M.D., Treas. F. A. BESLEY, M.D.

FACULTY

PATHOLOGY AND BACTERIOLOGY
F. R. Zeit, M.D.

MEDICINE
Arthur R. Elliott, A.M., M.D.
C. L. Mix, M.D.
Geo. F. Butler, M.D.
H. F. Goodwin, M.D.
W. A. Jaquith, M.D.

SURGERY
T. J. Sullivan, M.D.
Frederick A. Besley, M.D.
Wm. R. Cubbins, M.D.
A. E. Halsted, M.D.

ORTHOPEDIC SURGERY
Robert Hardon, M.D.

GYNECOLOGY
Franklin H. Martin, M.D.
Albert Goldspohn, M.D.
Emil Ries, M.D.
A. McDermid, M.B., M.D.

DISEASES OF RECTUM
Stuart Johnstone, M.D.

STOMACH AND INTESTINES
Fenton B. Turck, M.D.
Milton H. Mack, M.D.
G. F. Pierce, M.D.

EAR
A. H. Andrews, M.D.
C. S. Losey, M.D.
Randolph Brunson, M.D.

EYE
W. Franklin Coleman, M.D., M.R.C.S.
Geo. F. Suker, M.D.
Clark W. Hawley, M.D.
R. S. Patillo, M.D.

NOSE AND THROAT
G. P. Head, M.D.
O. J. Stein, M.D.
James T. Campbell, M.D.

NERVOUS DISEASES
Julius Grinker, M.D.

SPECIAL COURSES

In October we shall offer a General Course, lasting one month, beginning the first of the month, in which the student may make a selection from all the work of the School. This course includes General Medicine, General Surgery, Gynecology and Abdominal Surgery, Diseases of Children, Dermatology, Eye and Ear Diseases, Nose and Throat Diseases, Electro-Therapeutics and Obstetrics, all illustrated by Clinical teaching. Evening lectures on Anesthetics and Technique will also be a feature of the course (and the Student may, if he so desires, confine himself to any one of these departments).

Our faculty is so complete and our clinical material so abundant that we are able practically to conduct a SPECIAL SCHOOL in each department and the courses will consist of clinics and lectures extending throughout the entire day, so that every hour of the day may be profitably employed.

For catalogue and special literature, address,

FRANKLIN H. MARTIN, M.D., Secretary
2400 Dearborn Street, ... Chicago

FACULTY

OBSTETRICS
C. E. Paddock, M.D.
A. McDermid, M.D.

DISEASES OF CHILDREN
J. C. Cook, M.D.
Thos. Grant Allen, M.D.

SKIN AND VENEREAL DISEASES
W. L. Baum, M.D.

ANATOMY
R. C. Turck, M.D.

ELECTRO-PHYSICS
Noble M. Eberhart, M.D.

EXTRA-MURAL FACULTY

MEDICINE
Robert H. Babcock, M.D.
H. W. Gentles, M.D., C.M.

SURGERY
D. N. Eisendrath, M.D.
L. L. McArthur, M.D.
D. A. K. Steele, M.D.
J. B. Murphy, A.M., M.D.

GYNECOLOGY
Lester Frankenthal, M.D.
Henry T. Byford, M.D.
Henry P. Newman, M.D., A.M.

EAR
Norval H. Pierce, M.D.
Seth Scott Bishop, M.D., LL.D.

EYE
Casey A. Wood, M.D.
T. A. Woodruff, M.D.

NOSE AND THROAT
T. Melville Hardie, M.D., B.A.

NERVOUS DISEASES
Sydney Kuh, M.D.
Richard Dewey, M.D.
Daniel R. Brower, M.D.

SKIN AND VENEREAL DISEASES
L. Blake Baldwin, M.D.

10.1. Advertisement in the Journal of the American Medical Association *for the Post-Graduate Medical School of Chicago, which Martin had a prominent part in organizing.*

been practicing medicine for eight years and was the first significant example of Martin's incredible organizational and administrative skills.

The lower floors of the school were used for offices, classrooms, and the dispensary where indigent patients could receive free or inexpensive medical care. The upper floors were remodeled into a hospital, which later became the Chicago Charity Hospital. In Martin's assessment, the institution had "an aspect of thrift and academic activity.... We had a wholesome *esprit de corps*, for our faculty was interested and eager to follow our ideals of service...."[3] The equipment and facilities were modern and up to date, and "our downtown location was convenient to the hotels in which the visiting doctors—our prospective students—lived. Thus, we had a distinct advantage over our competitors."[3]

Within a month, students were enrolled, and patients were being seen in the outpatient dispensary. Dedicated members of the faculty were able to develop their clinical teaching skills. As Martin described it, "Ours was a 'show me' clinic, for the dispensary was well attended by patients who were available for purposes of demonstration," affording students the opportunity to learn important aspects of physical examination (Figure 10.1).[3] Dr. Besley characterized Martin's desire to establish the school as follows,

> This early thoughtful consideration of the need for the education of the actual workers in the field and his desire to help them was the motivating factor of his later activity in developing organizations for the elevation of the standards of surgery and the continuous education of all surgeons.[1]

Because of the school's popularity, a new building was designed and erected in downtown Chicago the following year and formally opened in mid-November 1890.[4] In the ensuing six years, the school continued to expand and improve, so another new, well-equipped building was erected at 2400 South Dearborn Street. The school occupied the seven-story building on September 1, 1896. It had surgical amphitheaters, electric lights and elevators, well-lighted laboratories and clinic rooms, and an amphitheater with a capacity for 250 students. One block from the Post-Graduate School they opened a thoroughly equipped surgical research and experimental laboratory, where students could operate on animals under faculty supervision. All medical schools subsequently installed this innovative type of laboratory.[5]

Elected Chairman of the AMA Section on Obstetrics and Diseases of Women at Age 37

Despite his protestations, Martin was unanimously elected Chairman of the Section on Obstetrics and Diseases of Women at the June 1894 meeting of the American Medical Association (AMA). In the process he learned about the circuitous procedures of organized medicine. He was unhappy with this first experience.[6] Later in his career he adapted well to working in the environment of medical politics as practiced by members of the American College of Surgeons (ACS) and the AMA.

Experiments on Ureteral Implantation into the Colon

Martin believed that, for patients whose ureters were blocked by an invading cancer such that urine could not flow into the urinary bladder, transection of the ureters would allow urine to flow from the kidneys and prevent renal failure. It would then be possible to re-implant the transected ureters into the small intestine or colon. The urine could then flow into the intestine where it would be partially reabsorbed, but the majority would be passed with bowel movements. The same procedure would be possible in younger patients with congenital exstrophy of the bladder, where the bladder opens onto the abdominal wall, and urine is excreted directly onto the abdominal wall. Martin surveyed the medical literature and found only one significant research effort on this topic and no evidence of the use of such a procedure in patients. In 1897 Martin said, "After several months of reading and rereading the existing literature, and carefully observing all of the pelvic organs in every patient upon whom I performed an abdominal operation, I decided to make an exhaustive study of the operative technique in our research laboratory."[7]

Initially, Martin and his assistants developed the technique for transecting and implanting the ureter into the colon in dogs. In most cases, the animals only survived a few days; at postmortem, the ureteral implantation site had successfully healed, but signs of infection were evident at other sites in the abdomen. Improving their antiseptic technique led to fewer intra-abdominal infections and improved survival in the dogs. Finally, Martin achieved success with several animals, and he was able to report his results. He did not report using the procedure in humans.[8] He presented his research findings and a review of the literature at the April 5, 1900, meeting of the Philadelphia Obstetrical Society. Because few physicians and surgeons in attendance had any significant experience with this formidable problem, he fielded many questions from the audience and thought the presentation went well.[9]

Martin was not a trained scientist and had no interest in pursuing a career in scientific research, but he did enjoy investigating a clinical problem. He said of the experience, "Obviously, I was not by training a scientist, for to my mind the application of scientific facts to a *practical accomplishment* was far more intriguing than the industrious and exclusive pursuit of a 'pure science' investigation."[9]

Once again, Martin had taken a medical conundrum from its identification to a solution entirely on his own—drawing on his discipline and ingenuity to forge ahead with a study when others might hesitate and miss the opportunity. The operation that Martin and his colleagues helped to perfect later became a mainstay of pelvic surgery.

Research on Ovarian Transplantation

In 1901, when Martin was 44 years old, a 29-year-old woman who'd had a bilateral oophorectomy during an operation for dysmenorrhea wrote Martin and several other surgeons, asking if it was possible to transplant ovaries so she could regain normal menstrual function and become pregnant. Once again, faced with a new clinical dilemma, Martin reviewed the medical literature. He discovered that a New York City surgeon, Robert T. Morris, had reported a series of human ovarian transplantations with supposed restoration of menstruation.[10] With this information, Martin developed in animals a technique for the procedure and informed the patient that he was prepared to proceed. One year later, the patient agreed to have the procedure. A short time later, a patient scheduled to have uterine surgery consented to donate a portion of her ovaries, and the operation was scheduled.

First Martin harvested one-third of both ovaries, along with a portion of the broad ligament from the patient donating her ovaries. The recipient, because her ovaries and fallopian tubes had been removed previously, did not have an opening for eggs to enter the uterus. Therefore, Martin created bilateral artificial openings in the uterus where an egg could theoretically enter the uterus. This was accomplished by making an incision in the uterus and suturing the mucous membrane of the uterus to the peritoneum on the exterior surface of the uterus. The patient's broad ligaments were incised close to the uterus and the ovaries sutured into this incision.[11] The technique did not involve revascularization of the transplanted ovary, which would be necessary for the tissue to survive. Even if the tissue had been revascularized, it would have undergone post-transplant rejection and ceased to function in a matter of days.

Postoperative monthly follow-up demonstrated some return of menstruation, but ultimately the procedure failed. Both the lack of a blood supply and rejection of the transplant would have prevented long-term functioning of the transplanted ovaries. Martin performed eight ovarian transplantations, but none of the patients developed normal menstruation. Despite the unsuccessful outcome, Martin's work and the efforts of others in this field set the stage for a better understanding of ovarian function and endocrinology in general.

Interestingly, Dr. Alexis Carrel, recipient of the 1912 Nobel Prize in Physiology or Medicine, contacted Martin to discuss his proposed experiments for transplanting ovaries in animals by anastomosing the ovarian vessels directly to the vessels of the animal receiving the transplant.[12]

Other "Research" Experience

As described in Chapter 5, Martin conducted a study during his internship in which he applied antiseptic techniques to the care of women on obstetrical wards who, to Martin's distress, frequently developed childbed (pueperal) fever and postpartum infections. Reviewing the medical literature, Martin learned that German scientists had shown that germs were responsible. More recent literature had revealed that the fingers of the patient's caregivers were the most likely source of these germs and the resultant infections. Martin concluded that the best way to avoid these infections was for the patient's caregivers to bathe their hands in 5 percent carbolic acid solution before examining their patients, which would markedly decrease the concentration of bacteria on their fingers and hands and hopefully significantly decrease the chance of infection.

In addition, the perineum would be made antiseptic by using Sir Joseph Lister's technique of bathing the area with carbolic acid. Martin used both practices in his study. Also, after delivery, the perineum was again bathed with carbolic acid and covered with a cloth soaked in carbolic acid solution. Martin treated 75 patients in this manner. The results were excellent. Of patients treated with antiseptic techniques, none died from infection and none developed childbed fever. Although he had no control group, just comparing his results to historical controls certainly would have proven the results significant.[13]

ACS historian Dr. David Nahrwold said, "Martin's boundless curiosity led him to conduct research on the treatment of uterine fibroids with galvanic current and, later, on ovarian transplantation."[14] After reviewing the experiments Martin completed, one gets the impression that he could have been an excellent research scientist. He had a knack for identifying a problem and designing a study to evaluate a possible solution. Regrettably, he did not have the training to design well-controlled studies that would yield statistically significant results. He had a high regard for the scientific approach to medical care, but he also believed that, ultimately, the best way to determine the appropriate operation for patients with a specific diagnosis was to observe master surgeons performing those procedures, and in the process gain insight into the difficulties they were experiencing performing some operations. Observation alone cannot teach surgeons the best procedure for a given diagnosis. Surgeons also need to know the results of clinical trials comparing different approaches to patient care and the results of scientific studies. Martin appeared to assume that most surgeons had already reviewed the relevant clinical and scientific literature before considering performing an operation and would therefore benefit from observing master surgeons.

REFERENCES

1. Besley, F. A. (1935). Franklin Martin—the surgeon. *Bull Am Coll Surg*, 20(2), 41.
2. Martin, F. H. (1933). *The Joy of Living: An Autobiography*, vol. 1 (pp. 303-305 and 308). New York, NY: Doubleday, Doran & Co.
3. Ibid., pp. 308-309.
4. Martin, F. H. (1933). *The Joy of Living: An Autobiography*, vol. 1 (pp. 310-312). New York, NY: Doubleday, Doran & Co.
5. Ibid., pp. 354-356.
6. Ibid., pp. 336-338.
7. Martin, F. H. (1933). *The Joy of Living: An Autobiography*, vol. 1 (pp. 364-368). New York, NY: Doubleday, Doran & Co.
8. Martin, F. H. (1899). Experimental implantation of ureters in the bowels. *Surg Gynecol & Obstet*, xiv, 307-310.
9. Martin, F. H. (1933). *The Joy of Living: An Autobiography*, vol. 1 (pp. 377-378). New York, NY: Doubleday, Doran & Co..
10. Morris, R. T. (1895). The ovarian graft. *New York Med J*, lxii, 436-437.
11. Martin, F. H. (1908). Transplantation of ovaries. *Surg Gynecol & Obstet*, vii, 7-21.
12. Martin, F. H. (1933). *The Joy of Living: An Autobiography*, vol. 1 (pp. 389-391). New York, NY: Doubleday, Doran & Co.
13. Ibid., pp. 214-216.
14. Nahrwold, D. L. (2016). *A Mirror Reflecting Surgery, Surgeons, and their College: The Bulletin of the American College of Surgeons* (p. 5). Chicago. IL: The American College of Surgeons.

Chapter 11

Founding of American College of Surgeons, SG&O, and Clinical Congress

oon noised ... those [illegible] thought ...
that the Corlins had ... on Sunday ...
... on the big bend. Every ...
claim on the big bend. Every ...
the raising on Saturday. Volunteer[s]
~~hands~~ were busy from all the neig[hbors] ...
the week, felling trees, hewing and adze ...
to shape for the new house. Early ...
g of Saturday a dozen or more ...
d boys were on hand to construct ...
ouse. A cellar had been dug in ...
... ready to be encased with ston[e] ...
... logs had been sunk in ...
eached a bed of solid clay beneath the ...
il, lumber had been brought from ...
w mill and a fine lot of dry ...
been contributed by generous neighbors ...
... ready to compete with ...
... steady oxen that had been brou[ght] ...
neighbors.

... by common cons[ent] ...
... for the day, no time ...
... all deviations came the great log ...
... chains about their necks a[nd] ...
... of the faithful oxen ...

Conceived, Developed, and Arranged for Publication of the Journal *Surgery, Gynecology and Obstetrics* in 1905

Martin (Figure 11.1) founded the journal *Surgery, Gynecology and Obstetrics (SG&O)* in July 1905 at age 48. At the time, most medical journals were financed and published by commercial firms. The only exception was the *Journal of the American Medical Association (JAMA)*, founded by Dr. Nathan S. Davis in 1883.

Commercial surgical journals were poorly edited and practicing surgeons were minimally involved in reviewing submitted manuscripts. This left practicing surgeons without a noncommercial journal in which to publish their articles and to use as a source of information about improvements in the practice of clinical surgery. Martin believed "that this unfortunate condition could be remedied if the profession were to organize a practical journal for practical surgeons, edited by active surgeons instead of *littérateurs* only remotely connected with clinical work."[1] He conceived, developed, and arranged for such a publication, *SG&O*, which remains in publication today as the *Journal of the American College of Surgeons (JACS)*.

Martin arranged for a friend and reliable publisher, Mr. T. E. Donnelley of R. R. Donnelley & Sons of Chicago, to publish the journal. This was to be his administrative style throughout his career: if he saw a problem, he evaluated it, and if he decided it required action, he went forward. Although he might seek advice, he almost never brought in others until he had decided on a solution. This method differs from that of many leaders, both in the past and today, who appoint large committees to evaluate problems and make recommendations before a decision is made—a process that may take from months to years to run its course.

Martin discussed his proposal with Dr. John B. Murphy (Figure 11.2), a long-time friend, and other surgeons. With their encouragement, he decided to proceed with the project himself, although he had not initially planned to take on the administrative tasks as he "was not seeking

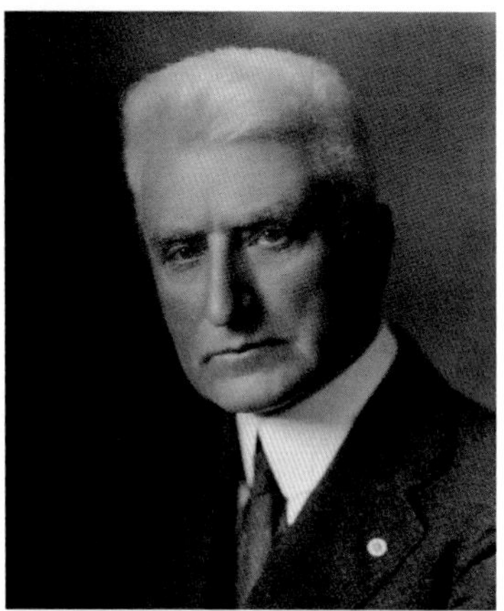

11.1. Dr. Martin's official ACS portrait from the 1920s.

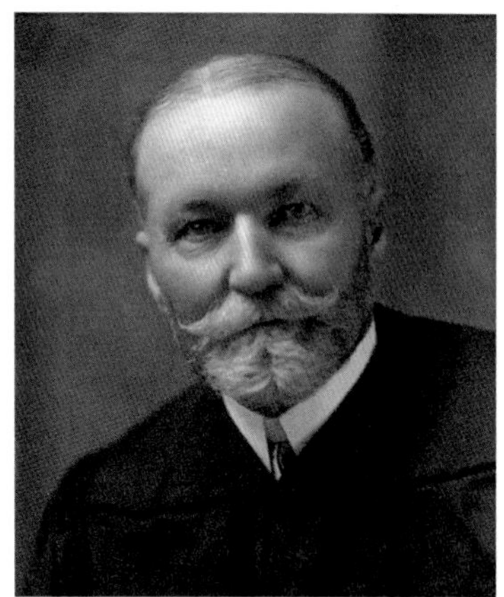

11.2. Dr. John B. Murphy, another famous Chicago surgeon raised in rural Wisconsin.

another job."[1] Dr. Murphy was especially enthusiastic, telling Martin that this was a job Martin could and should do. Dr. Murphy indicated he and other surgeons would help finance the project, but the journal should be under Martin's control.

Although at first Martin was unenthusiastic about becoming the journal's editor, eventually he decided that Dr. Murphy was right: this was a job he should do. Martin's secretary, Margaret Bowen, whose judgment he respected, also encouraged him to take on this new responsibility. As discussed in Chapter 7, his wife, Isabelle, initially was opposed to the idea because she felt he already was working long hours. Eventually she yielded to his strong desire to proceed with the new enterprise. Martin enlisted the help of four young surgeon friends—Frederic A. Besley, Allen B. Kanavel, William R. Cubbins, and John Hollister—to be members of the Editorial Staff (Figure 11.3). Martin made the point that only actual practitioners of surgery, not littérateurs, were to serve on the Editorial Board and the Editorial Staff.

Financial backing for *SG&O* was solicited from interested surgeons, but Martin and his wife kept a controlling 51 percent interest.

Dr. Nicholas Senn of Chicago, who when he lived in Milwaukee had signed Martin's Wisconsin State Medical Society credentials establishing Martin's eligibility to matriculate to medical school in Chicago, was named Chief of the Editorial Board and authored the lead article in

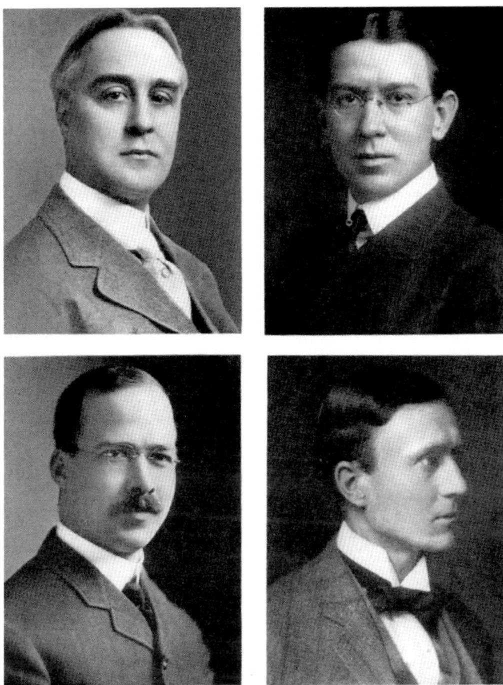

11.3. The four young surgeons who assisted in the initial planning for the publication of Surgery, Gynecology & Obstetrics *(clockwise from top left): Frederic A. Besley, Allen B. Kanavel, William R. Cubbins, and John Hollister.*

the first issue. The Editorial Board comprised 11 prestigious Chicago surgeons, and Drs. George W. Crile, William Mayo, Charles Mayo, John B. Murphy, and Albert J. Ochsner, among other surgical leaders, were listed as collaborators. Martin guided the journal from conception to publication, with 600 initial subscriptions, in just six months (Figure 11.4). Over the next few years, the journal grew and became a tremendous success professionally, scientifically, and financially. To this day *JACS* remains one of the world's premier surgical journals.[1]

SG&O established a popular British edition in 1908, with an editorial staff from the British Empire, and in 1913 added the *International Abstracts of Surgery*, which included abstracts from the surgical literature from around the world and an up-to-date bibliography of the current surgical literature. These two additions doubled the size of the journal and added to its prestige.[1]

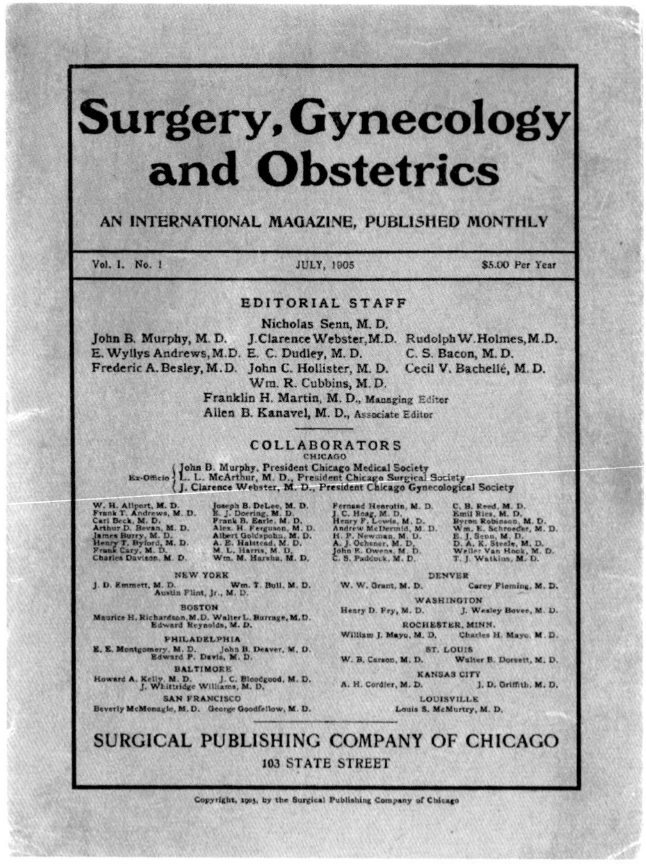

Surgery, Gynecology and Obstetrics

AN INTERNATIONAL MAGAZINE, PUBLISHED MONTHLY

Vol. I. No. 1 JULY, 1905 $5.00 Per Year

EDITORIAL STAFF

Nicholas Senn, M. D.
John B. Murphy, M. D. J. Clarence Webster, M.D. Rudolph W. Holmes, M.D.
E. Wyllys Andrews, M.D. E. C. Dudley, M. D. C. S. Bacon, M. D.
Frederic A. Besley, M.D. John C. Hollister, M. D. Cecil V. Bachellé, M. D.
Wm. R. Cubbins, M. D.
Franklin H. Martin, M. D., Managing Editor
Allen B. Kanavel, M. D., Associate Editor

COLLABORATORS

CHICAGO

Ex-Officio { John B. Murphy, President Chicago Medical Society
L. L. McArthur, M. D., President Chicago Surgical Society
J. Clarence Webster, M. D., President Chicago Gynecological Society }

W. H. Allport, M. D. · Frank T. Andrews, M. D. · Carl Beck, M. D. · Arthur D. Bevan, M. D. · James Burry, M. D. · Henry T. Byford, M. D. · Frank Cary, M. D. · Charles Davison, M. D.

Joseph B. DeLee, M. D. · E. J. Doering, M. D. · Frank B. Earle, M. D. · Alex. H. Ferguson, M. D. · Albert Goldspohn, M. D. · A. E. Halstead, M. D. · M. L. Harris, M. D. · Wm. M. Harsha, M. D.

Fernand Henrotin, M. D. · J. C. Hoag, M. D. · Henry F. Lewis, M. D. · Andrew McDermid, M. D. · H. P. Newman, M. D. · A. J. Ochsner, M. D. · John E. Owens, M. D. · C. S. Paddock, M. D.

C. B. Reed, M. D. · Emil Ries, M. D. · Byron Robinson, M. D. · Wm. E. Schroeder, M. D. · E. J. Senn, M. D. · D. A. K. Steele, M. D. · Weller Van Hook, M. D. · T. J. Watkins, M. D.

NEW YORK
J. D. Emmett, M. D. Wm. T. Bull, M. D.
Austin Flint, Jr., M. D.

BOSTON
Maurice H. Richardson, M.D. Walter L. Burrage, M.D.
Edward Reynolds, M. D.

PHILADELPHIA
E. E. Montgomery, M. D. John B. Deaver, M. D.
Edward P. Davis, M. D.

BALTIMORE
Howard A. Kelly, M. D. J. C. Bloodgood, M. D.
J. Whittridge Williams, M. D.

SAN FRANCISCO
Beverly McMonagle, M. D. George Goodfellow, M. D.

DENVER
W. W. Grant, M. D. Carey Fleming, M. D.

WASHINGTON
Henry D. Fry, M. D. J. Wesley Bovee, M. D.

ROCHESTER, MINN.
William J. Mayo, M. D. Charles H. Mayo, M. D.

ST. LOUIS
W. B. Carson, M. D. Walter B. Dorsett, M. D.

KANSAS CITY
A. H. Cordier, M. D. J. D. Griffith, M. D.

LOUISVILLE
Louis S. McMurtry, M. D.

SURGICAL PUBLISHING COMPANY OF CHICAGO
103 STATE STREET

Copyright, 1905, by the Surgical Publishing Company of Chicago

11.4. Volume 1, Number 1, of Surgery, Gynecology & Obstetrics. *Note the number of prominent surgeons listed on the editorial staff and as contributors.*

Conceived and Developed Format for the Clinical Congress of Surgeons of North America in 1910

Encouraged by the success of *SG&O,* in 1910, at age 53, Martin conceived of an annual clinical congress for surgeons. He believed that inadequately trained but dedicated young surgeons who were anxious to learn would profit from visits to the clinics of outstanding surgeons and from the opportunity to hear presentations from successful practitioners. Martin believed that "it was far better to have a practicing surgeon demonstrate his work than to have him tell about it."[2]

Martin believed that practicing surgeons were dissatisfied with presentations made by "non-practicing editors who acted merely as interpreters"[2] and were seeking opportunities to observe master surgeons performing operations as a way to better understand the technical and mechanical problems they might encounter when performing procedures and possible solutions. Martin believed that only observation allowed a surgeon to decide which procedures were worthwhile. At this point in his career, Martin believed in the importance of clinical and scientific studies when considering appropriate therapies for patients; but when determining which operation was the best procedure for patients, observing master surgeons was an equally important aspect of the final decision.

An already established organization—the Society of Clinical Surgery—offered programs where its members visited large surgical centers to observe their colleagues performing operations. But participation was limited to active members of the group, who were few in number. The annual clinical congress that Martin envisioned would be open to all interested surgeons, and after further consideration he outlined the format for such a gathering. The first meeting was announced in an editorial in the September 1910 issue of *SG&O*. The announcement discussed the increased popularity of learning surgical technique through direct observation of master surgeons, and invited all physicians in the U.S. and Canada who were interested in surgery to observe operations at large Chicago medical centers. A committee of enthusiastic Chicago surgeons was organized to work out the meeting details.

In November 1910, the first Clinical Congress of Surgeons of North America took place in Chicago. The Congress, which lasted two weeks, was composed of daytime operative clinics and evening paper presentations. It was overwhelmingly well received. Two hundred surgeons were expected, but 1,300 attended. Many of the clinics were filled beyond capacity. As Martin described it, "The men in attendance were discriminating. They wanted to see many modest operators whose work had attracted them but who were not prominent in the regular society proceeding; men who were proving themselves in action."[2]

On the last day of the Congress, at the request of an attendee, a meeting was convened to plan a permanent organization for future congresses. The second Congress took place in 1911 in Philadelphia and was equally successful. Fifteen hundred physicians registered and probably an equal number participated without registering. With some changes in format, the Clinical Congress continues today as the Clinical Congress of the American College of Surgeons.[2]

A New Surgical Organization, the American College of Surgeons

While traveling to New York City for the third annual Clinical Congress of Surgeons in 1912, at age 55, Martin outlined the format for a new surgical organization to unite U.S. and Canadian surgeons in a single association. The new group would be closely allied with and use the organizational structure of the Clinical Congress. Martin later wrote, "The plan was dictated to the train stenographer, and the result placed in my pocket, that it might 'age' while I indulged in more mature thought."[3] On arrival in New York, he contacted Dr. John B. Murphy to discuss the formation of this new organization, which would have defined qualifications for membership and would have the following goals:

- A standard of professional, ethical, and moral requirements for every authorized graduate of medicine who practices general surgery or any of its specialties
- A supplementary degree for operating surgeons
- Special letters to indicate fellowship in the college
- A published list of members
- The appointment of a committee of 12 members of the Clinical Congress with full power to proceed with the plan

Dr. Murphy was interested and supportive of the plan to develop this new organization, the American College of Surgeons (ACS). Martin next presented the proposal to Dr. Edward Martin, President of the Clinical Congress of Surgeons of North America, and received his endorsement.

At the business meeting of the 1912 Clinical Congress, Martin presented his plan and moved for its adoption. Dr. Murphy seconded

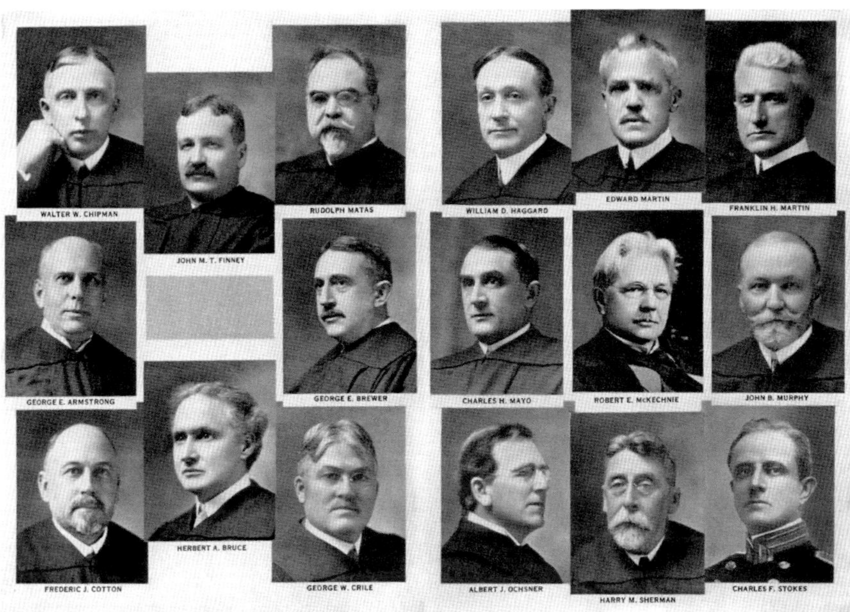

11.5. Original Board of Regents of the American College of Surgeons.

the motion and gave a powerful speech recommending its approval. The motion was approved unanimously, and an organizing committee was appointed that included several prominent surgeons, including Drs. Murphy, Rudolph Matas, Albert J. Ochsner, Charles Mayo, John M. T. Finney, George W. Crile, Edward Martin, and Franklin Martin.

At the first meeting of the organizing committee, Martin proposed that he visit major cities in Canada and the U.S. to present the plan for the new organization to an assembly of surgeons in each of those cities. Over the next few months Martin traveled North America promoting the new college. At many of these meetings, attendees expressed opposition to the new organization—for reasons including that it would amount to a union, that it would be undemocratic, that universities or the American Medical Association could fill the same role—but overall, the meetings were successful, and many of the surgeons agreed to attend the organizational meeting in Washington, DC, in December.[3]

Although other organizations had discussed forming a national college of surgeons, none had followed through. It took Martin's organizational skills and confidence to make the formation of such a society possible. Dr. William Mayo said of Martin's founding of the ACS:

"Dr. Martin, with broad vision, wished to develop an association which would have for its purpose the better care of the American people...."[3]

Martin and his cofounders developed surgical training standards and created a list of minimum standards for surgeons in independent practice. The College would recognize surgeons who met the standards. Finally, on November 15, 1913, the organizational meeting was convened, with 450 surgeons attending. The charter and bylaws were presented and unanimously approved. The first Board of Directors was elected (Figure 11.5).[3] The nominating committee proposed the following: for President, Dr. John M. T. Finney, of Johns Hopkins University; for Vice-Presidents, Dr. Walter H. Chipman and Dr. Rudolf Matas; for General Secretary, Dr. Franklin H. Martin; and for Treasurer, Dr. Albert J. Ochsner. For political reasons, and because many of the physicians present were suspicious of the motives of the Chicago surgeons and of their desire to have control of the College, it was important that the first president not be from Chicago. Therefore Dr. Finney's nomination was well received. The American College of Surgeons was created.

The only other significant item of business was brought forth by Dr. Miles F. Porter of Indiana. It was "a plea for a declaration against the division of fees, the paying of commissions for surgical work, and buying and selling of patients."[3] A formal declaration against this practice was adopted. Martin said, "The first official gun had been fired by the new College against an abomination in the economics of medicine—fee division." He celebrated this accomplishment as an important first move by the College.[3]

Dr. Frederic A. Besley later said of Martin's founding of the College,

> As a result of his great vision, his courage, his indomitable will to succeed, and his unusual ability as an organizer, he has [built] the American College of Surgeons which will endure in perpetuity as a monument to his understanding of the need for continuous surgical teaching in its broadest sense.[5]

Dr. George W. Crile said,

> ...there was no one man who could have equaled the performance of Franklin Martin as Director-General, for more than to any other one man, the credit belongs to him for the

> foundation of the College, its organization, ...the shaping of its policies, the solving of the many difficult executive problems which have repeatedly presented themselves.[6]

In the short span of eight years, Franklin Martin had conceived, developed, and founded almost single-handedly the journal *SG&O*, the Clinical Congress of Surgeons of North America, and the American College of Surgeons. Martin later said,

> These organizations have suggested standards for surgery and for the betterment of hospitals, and they have promoted a partnership between the general public and the scientific profession which has resulted in wholesome and mutual understanding and cooperation.[7]

To some, it may seem inconceivable that a man who spent the first 20 years of his life as a farm laborer would have the strength of character, discipline, and confidence to accomplish all of this with minimal help from other surgeons. I believe it was because of his rural upbringing that he had developed those qualities.

References

1. Martin, F. H. (1933). *The Joy of Living: An Autobiography,* vol. 1 (pp. 397-401). New York, NY: Doubleday, Doran & Co.
2. Ibid., pp. 402-408.
3. Ibid., pp. 409-431.
4. Mayo, W. J. Foreword. In: Martin, F. H. (1933). *The Joy of Living: An Autobiography,* vol. 1 (p. xi). New York, NY: Doubleday, Doran & Co.
5. Besley, F. A. (1935). Franklin H. Martin—the surgeon. *Bull Am Coll Surg,* 20(2), 43.
6. Crile, G. (1935). Franklin H. Martin and The American College of Surgeons. *Bull Am Coll Surg,* 20(2), 51.
7. Martin, F. H. (1933). *The Joy of Living: An Autobiography,* vol. 1 (p. viii). New York, NY: Doubleday, Doran & Co.

Chapter 12

Establishment of Hospital Standards

...oon houses ... that the Corliss house ... had brought ... invitations on Sunday had ... Every ... claim on the big hand. ... the raising on Saturday. Volunteers ... were busy from all the neigh... the week, felling trees, hewing and adzing ... the shape for the new house. Early ... of Saturday a dozen or more ... and boys were on hand to construct ... house. A cellar had been dug in ... ready to be encased with stone ... logs had been sunk in ... reached a bed of solid clay beneath the ... lumber had been brought from ... saw mill and a fine lot of ... been contributed by generous neighbors ... ready to compete with ... that had been ... Sunday oxen ... neighbors ... In no instance by common consent ... of the yeomen for the day. No time was ... all directions came the great logs ... chains about their necks ... by the faithful oxen ...

ESTABLISHMENT OF HOSPITAL STANDARDS

The idea of a hospital standardization program was first introduced to surgeons at the November 15, 1912, business meeting of the Clinical Congress of Surgeons of North America in New York. After Martin's proposal to create the American College of Surgeons (ACS) was approved at the Clinical Congress, Dr. Allen B. Kanavel, a young associate of Martin's, presented a resolution supporting the standardization of hospital work and equipment. This passed and a committee was formed under the auspices of the Clinical Congress with Dr. Ernest Codman as chairman. Dr. Codman was a Boston surgeon with an ardent interest in improving the quality of hospital care. He was the originator of the "end-result system," whereby "Surgeons and hospitals would monitor and improve their clinical outcomes through long-term follow-up of their patients."[1] Reading Martin's thoughts on hospital standardization, it is obvious that Dr. Kanavel proposed this resolution with Martin's support.

Improving the clinical practice of medicine was part of the original stated purposes of the ACS, and Martin believed that it would be easier to accomplish such improvement in well-organized and well-equipped hospitals. Because Codman's committee had not produced any tangible results in more than two years, Codman resigned, and the committee disbanded at the Clinical Congress in 1915. The function of the committee was then assumed by the College.[2]

The case records submitted by applicants for membership in the ACS indicated that many surgeons were practicing in hospitals that lacked the facilities essential for high-quality, science-based patient care. In these hospitals, laboratory facilities were deficient, medical staffs were unorganized, and cases were not systematically recorded and reviewed. When applicants were refused admission to the ACS because of unacceptable case records, hospitals requested clarification of the College's hospital standards. Specifically, they wanted elaboration about appropriate record forms, laboratory standards, and staff organization standards.[3]

The College decided it was time to clarify the standards they expected hospitals to meet, and the first conference on hospital standardization took place October 19–20, 1917, in Chicago. In his introductory statement at the conference Martin said,

> We have no compulsory power over hospitals that do not enter into the program with us. But we have with us the strong support of some 4,000 Fellows and the force of public opinion because what we want is right. Let me say that the standardization of hospitals covering a continent can be accomplished only by firmness and by the untiring exercise of the courage of our convictions. Let me urge also that swiftness of action inspires confidence and defeats opposition.[4]

At the same conference, Dr. John A. Hornsby, editor of *The Modern Hospital,* gave a bleak assessment of the overall quality of U.S. hospitals. In Dr. Hornsby's assessment, the patient record in 75 percent of American hospitals was "practically valueless." Frequently, an admitting diagnosis was omitted from the record and there was no examination at the time of admission. In 75 percent of hospitals, even surgery patients did not have a diagnosis listed in the record before their operation. X rays often were obtained by untrained personnel and were not interpreted until the consulting radiologist spent a day at the hospital.[5]

After hearing this type of information at the conference, Dr. John G. Bowman, ACS Director, immediately created a short list of factors that he considered "imperative in any hospital for the proper care of patients."[6] They were as follows:

- Case records for all patients
- Laboratory facilities capable of performing studies essential in the diagnosis and treatment of patients admitted for care under normal conditions
- Cooperation between the hospital authorities and hospital physicians to prohibit the practice of division of fees

Dr. Bowman believed that these factors were only a beginning and that other areas would require attention in the future.[6]

Following the conference, the College leadership spent two years analyzing hospitals to establish the overall quality of the care provided in the U.S. In October 1919, at the annual Clinical Congress in New York City, Dr. Bowman reported on this analysis. In a survey of 671 hospitals with 100 or more beds, only 198 (30 percent) were in full compliance with the College's minimum standard for hospitals. Only 264 (39 percent) had staff meetings, in only 301 (45 percent) were physical examinations conducted before treatment, and in only 291 (43 percent) did progress notes appear in the record.[7]

On a more positive note, in 466 hospitals (69 percent) a final diagnosis was included in the patient's record at the time of discharge from the hospital, and in 442 hospitals (66 percent) laboratory, pathology, and/or X-ray findings were included in the patient's record.[7] One year later, at a follow-up review, the percentage of fully compliant hospitals had risen from 30 percent to 58 percent, demonstrating the impact of the College's program—thus improving the status of the program and the reputation of the College.[8]

At the end of this analysis, the ACS Regents decided to create a set of minimum hospital standards designed to safeguard patients by requiring the following:

- That all physicians working in the hospital be competent and worthy in character and in matters of professional ethics
- That physicians be organized as a medical staff
- That the staff, with the approval of the governing board of the hospital, adopt a set of rules, regulations, and policies governing their professional work
- That clinical and pathological laboratories be adequate to ensure a correct diagnosis
- That each patient's medical record be accurate and include a thorough evaluation of the patient's symptoms and a diagnosis
- That there be monthly staff meetings where patient care would be audited
- That there be no evidence of division of fees

This list of safeguards was codified and published by the ACS in "The Minimum Standard" for hospitals.[7]

Although acceptance of the standards was voluntary, by the early 1930s more than 2,000 hospitals had been surveyed and approved. This program, as administered by the College, had the support of the public and organizations interested in high-quality hospital care. Among the more important benefits of the program were a significant reduction in length of stay, a decrease in infection and complication rates, and lower mortality rates. Through the years, minimum standards were established for multiple hospital functions, including operating room design and management, casualty services (emergency room), trauma services, care of patients with fractures, physical therapy services, performance of autopsies, nursing services, dietary services, social services, performance of anesthesia, and treatment of infected wounds.[9]

Of interest, during a 1924 visit to Australia and New Zealand, Dr. William Mayo and Martin were asked to discuss in detail the College's hospital standards program. Two years later, in 1926, Dr. Malcolm T. MacEachern, Director of the College's Department of Hospital Standardization, traveled to Australia and New Zealand at their governments' request to survey their facilities and assist in instituting the Minimum Standard of the College in their hospitals.[10]

The development and promulgation of the hospital standards program by the ACS under Martin's supervision was a phenomenally successful endeavor that had a significant impact on the quality of patient care provided in hospitals throughout the U.S., Canada, and other countries. The College was at no time obligated to finance and administer the program, but under Martin it did so with tremendous vigor.

Martin and the College Regents perceived a need and took on the responsibility of addressing that need. Ultimately it was Martin's program.[3] It is my judgment that this program should be included in the list of Martin's major accomplishments, for without his leadership it would not have developed into the tremendously successful program it became. With his other major accomplishments—founding the College, *SG&O*, and the Clinical Congress—Martin had minimal organizational backing, and therefore he had to proceed using his personal organizational skills, exceptional leadership skills, and resourcefulness; whereas with the hospital standardization program he was able to use the College structure to establish and promote the program.

In 1951, after almost 35 years of continuous financial support and management of the hospital standardization program, the College—following a year-long series of meetings with the American Medical Association, the American Hospital Association, the American College of Physicians, and the Canadian Medical Association—agreed to the formation of a new entity, the Joint Commission on the Accreditation of Hospitals (JCAHO), which would assume responsibility for the hospital standardization program. JCAHO (later The Joint Commission) became functional in January 1952.[11]

The College initially had assumed sole financial responsibility for the program because ACS leadership thought that hospitals would withdraw from the program if they had to pay a fee. At the time the ACS turned the hospital standardization program over to JCAHO, it had spent more than $2 million on the program—an expense it could no longer afford.[12]

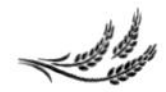

REFERENCES

1. Nahrwold, D. L., Kernahan, P. J. (2012). *A Century of Surgeons and Surgery: The American College of Surgeons 1913–2012* (pp. 11-12). Chicago, IL: American College of Surgeons.
2. Ibid., pp. 33-34.
3. Martin, F. H. (1933). *The Joy of Living: An Autobiography*, vol. 1 (pp. 445-447). New York, NY: Doubleday, Doran & Co.
4. Martin, F. H. (1917). Statement of Secretary General. *Bull Am Coll Surg*, 3(1), 3.
5. Hornsby, J. (1917). The hospital problem of today—what is it? *Bull Am Coll Surg*, 3(1), 4-11.
6. Bowman, J. G. (1918). Standard of efficiency for the first hospital survey of the College. *Bull Am Coll Surg*, 3(3), 1-7.
7. Bowman, J. G. (1920). The minimum standard. *Bull Am Coll Surg*, 4(3), 3-6.
8. Bowman, J. G., (1920). General hospitals of 100 or more beds: Report for 1919. *Bull Am Coll Surg*, 4(4), 3-5.

9. Martin, F. H. (1928). Report on hospital standardization for the year 1927. *Bull Am Coll Surg*, 12(1), 3-30.
10. Martin, F. H. (1933). *The Joy of Living: An Autobiography*, vol. 1 (pp. 453-455). New York, NY: Doubleday, Doran & Co.
11. Nahrwold, D. L., Kernahan, P. J. (2012). *A Century of Surgeons and Surgery: The American College of Surgeons 1913–2012* (pp. 204-206). Chicago, IL: American College of Surgeons.
12. Nahrwold, D. L. (2015). *A Mirror Reflecting Surgery, Surgeons, and their College: The Bulletin of the American College of Surgeons* (p. 478-479). Chicago, IL: The American College of Surgeons.

Chapter 13

Martin and World War I: Outbreak, Preparation, and Participation

you moved ov [illegible]
that the Corliss house thought
Cession on Sunday had . Every bo
claim on the big bend.
the raising on Saturday. Volunteer
[illegible] were busy from all the neig adjoin
the week, felling trees, hewing and [illegible]
ch shop for the new house. Early
g of Saturday a dozen or more st
and boys were on hand to construc
ouse. A cellar had been dug in t
[illegible] ready to be encased with sto
alim logs had been sunk in ben
eached a bed of solid clay beneath th
il, lumber had been brought from
aw mill and a fine lot of dry
been contributed by generous neighbors
on [illegible] ready to compete with Su
that had been bro
inday oxen
neighbors.
Your brother by common con
of the game
mon for the day. No time over
the great logs
all directions came their necks a
iron chains about their necks and
of the faithful oxen

Daring Rescue of Inez Stone from Munich

As the 1914 Clinical Congress of Surgeons of North America, held in London, England, was ending on August 1, World War I broke out when Germany declared war on Russia. Shortly thereafter, Germany also declared war on France and Belgium, and Britain declared war on Germany. This situation effectively stranded 1,100 surgeons and their families in London with no easily identifiable means of traveling home. Isabelle's niece, Inez Stone, who had traveled with the Martins to England, was in Munich, Germany, visiting friends and hadn't been in contact with her family for several days. At Dr. Frank Simpson's insistence, he and Martin left almost immediately to attempt the rescue of Ms. Stone. Dr. Simpson, an influential and close friend of Martin's, was a gynecologist and abdominal surgeon from Pittsburgh when Martin met him in 1909. He was an energetic member of the American Gynecological Society, of which he was president in 1915. His contributions to the medical literature were numerous and valuable. He was admired for his strength of character and his uncompromising defense of the highest traditions of the profession of surgery.

After crossing the channel and traveling to Paris, Martin and Simpson were unable to proceed to Germany because all trains headed east were reserved for the mobilization of French Army personnel, so they returned to London.

On their return to London, they became aware of a new committee that had been formed by a small group of New York bankers, the Committee for the Relief of Stranded Americans, that was planning an organizational meeting. Martin described the poorly organized effort, "Frank and I found, however, that there was neither a formulated program nor a leader. We realized that without leadership there would be confusion if not real trouble."[1] Martin and Simpson met with the leaders of the group and helped devise a plan for the meeting. One of the bankers, Mr. Theodore Hetzler, was selected to chair the meeting.

Martin personally called the meeting to order and introduced Mr. Hetzler. Martin's and Simpson's assistance contributed to the formation of an organization that could efficiently assist the stranded Americans.

Another major problem was the difficulties many Americans were having obtaining money on letters of credit. Martin and Simpson arranged through Thos. Cook & Son for the Americans to obtain small amounts of cash for expenses.

Unlike their fellow Clinical Congress attendees and other stranded Americans, Martin and Simpson didn't just vent their frustrations. They did what resourceful, commanding leaders do: identify solutions and act.

With these problems under control, Martin returned to the task of rescuing Inez Stone. He met and pooled resources with Mr. John Morrow of New York and Chicago, whose wife and sister-in-law also were stranded in Munich. Together they were able to secure the assistance of Mr. Geheimrat S. Bergeman, a wealthy and influential German whom Morrow had met earlier. Because they could not travel to Germany through France, they crossed the English Channel to the Netherlands and traveled by train to the German border. After crossing the border into Germany, they continued their often delayed and frustrating journey to Munich, again by train. Because of the slowness of the train through Germany, Mr. Bergeman arranged for a chauffeur-driven automobile to continue the journey. Their whirlwind, often heart-pounding trip took them through German towns that were mobilizing for war. Their intrepid chauffeur, Gerhardt, cadged rationed gasoline on numerous occasions. After leaving them in Cologne, Mr. Bergeman used his influence to ease the logistics for the remainder of their journey. On arrival in Munich, Martin was easily reunited with Inez and likewise Mr. Morrow with his wife. Martin made plans to return to London two days hence while Morrow made plans to return to America directly from Germany. On the return trip to London, Inez used her excellent German and soothing presence to persuade people of their innocent intent, and they boldly proceeded through military traffic by flying a German flag—which, unbeknownst to them, was only to be flown by the military and the royal family. The remainder of the trip through Germany, Holland, and across the English Channel went smoothly, and they reached London on August 20. The following day they began planning their return home.[1]

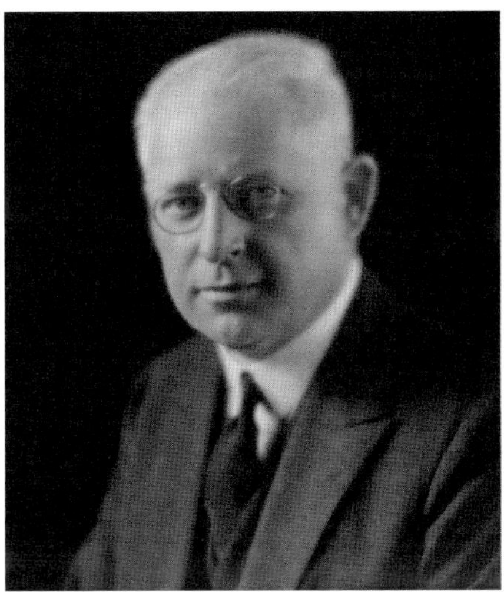

13.1. Dr. Frank Simpson.

By his description, Martin obviously relished the adventure. The entire enterprise was detailed in an August 22, 1914, article in the *New York Times* and in a recent article in the *Bulletin of the American College of Surgeons.*[2,3]

The tremendous risk Martin took traveling to Munich to rescue his wife's niece truly was an act of altruism and grit, yet he did it without a second thought—just another example from a different realm demonstrating how Martin proceeded deliberately once he had outlined a plan of action, despite the risks to his personal safety. The well-being and safety of Inez were all that mattered to him.

ORGANIZATION OF THE COMMITTEE OF AMERICAN PHYSICIANS FOR MEDICAL PREPAREDNESS BY DR. FRANK SIMPSON WITH MARTIN'S ASSISTANCE

In early 1916, prior to the United States' entry into World War I, Dr. Frank Simpson (Figure 13.1), with the encouragement and support of Martin, formed the Committee of American Physicians for Medical Preparedness to make ready American medicine for the war effort. The committee was created with support from the American Medical Association, the American Surgical Association, the Congress of Physicians and Surgeons of North America, the Clinical Congress of Surgeons of North America, and the American College of Surgeons. Simpson stressed that the organizational structure of the committee must be comprehensive and include all facets of medical care. The national medical and surgical associations were asked to participate in developing a medical preparedness plan so that they would be available and prepared to support the military if the U.S. entered the war. Many of the invitees already supported such preparations.

The initial, organizational meeting occurred April 14, 1916, and included many prominent physicians: William and Charles Mayo, George W. Crile, John B. Murphy, Albert J. Ochsner, Edward Martin, Frank Billings, and, of course, Franklin Martin and Frank Simpson. The Surgeons General of the Army, Navy, and Public Health Service were ex-officio members of the committee. To help identify the country's medical resources, advisory committees were appointed from each state.

On April 20, 1916, in a meeting with President Woodrow Wilson, the committee offered its assistance to the government. President Wilson forwarded the offer to the Secretaries of the Army, Navy, and American Red Cross with a positive recommendation. From this point forward Dr. Simpson, as committee secretary, was in frequent contact with the Secretary of War Newton D. Baker and the Secretary of the Navy Josephus Daniels, in addition to the Surgeons General of the Army, General William C. Gorgas; the Navy, Rear Admiral William C. Braisted; and the Public Health Service, Rupert Blue; as well as the Director-General of Military Relief for the American Red Cross, Colonel Jefferson R. Kean.

Drs. Simpson and Martin formed the committee at a time when it seemed to them that the leaders of the executive branch of the government were inadequately prepared for the distinct possibility of the nation joining the war. Drs. Simpson and Martin, two like-minded individuals, were convinced of the absolute necessity of their plan. Martin said of his interactions with Simpson: "Repeatedly, before the United States entered the struggle, he would say to me: 'Professor, we must arouse the doctors to prepare for what will soon be our war.'"[4] Martin's description of Simpson, as follows, was remarkably similar to the way others described him,

> Though he was feared, he commanded the respect of those who opposed the advancement of his progressive ideas. A conservative

> in thought, he was radical and determined in action. His plans were carefully conceived and thoroughly and industriously executed. Caution and vigilance were paramount.[4]

You couldn't easily compose a more accurate description of Martin himself, and it is no surprise how fast and true their rapport was. Martin said of his relationship with Simpson,

> Into the lives of all of us come individuals who influence us profoundly and who create for us epochs of unusual importance. In the earlier contacts they may be casual acquaintances who socially and professionally attract us; but association begets admiration, and their characters, minds, and manner of action develop mutual sympathies and weld strong friendships whose highest expression is co-operative action.[4]

It was a perfect description of their relationship during the founding of the committee and throughout the war effort.[4]

Martin Appointed to the Advisory Commission of the Council of National Defense

Although most U.S. citizens were opposed to the country entering World War I, even in 1916 it seemed inevitable, and in the summer of 1916 Congress passed a bill providing for a Council of National Defense with a civilian Advisory Commission in preparation for the eventuality of the U.S. entering the war. These bodies were founded to act as a direct channel for communication between American business and science and the federal government, especially the President. The Advisory Commission was designed to deal with all aspects of national defense. Initially the medical profession did not have a seat on the Advisory Commission, but after extensive lobbying by Dr. Simpson, one of the seven positions on the Commission was reserved for medicine. After the bill passed on August 29, 1916, Simpson declared to Martin that he, Martin, must be appointed to the Commission. Martin argued that Simpson was a better choice because he was well known in Washington, he already had a plan of action for medical preparedness, and the Commission would expect his appointment. Despite Mar-

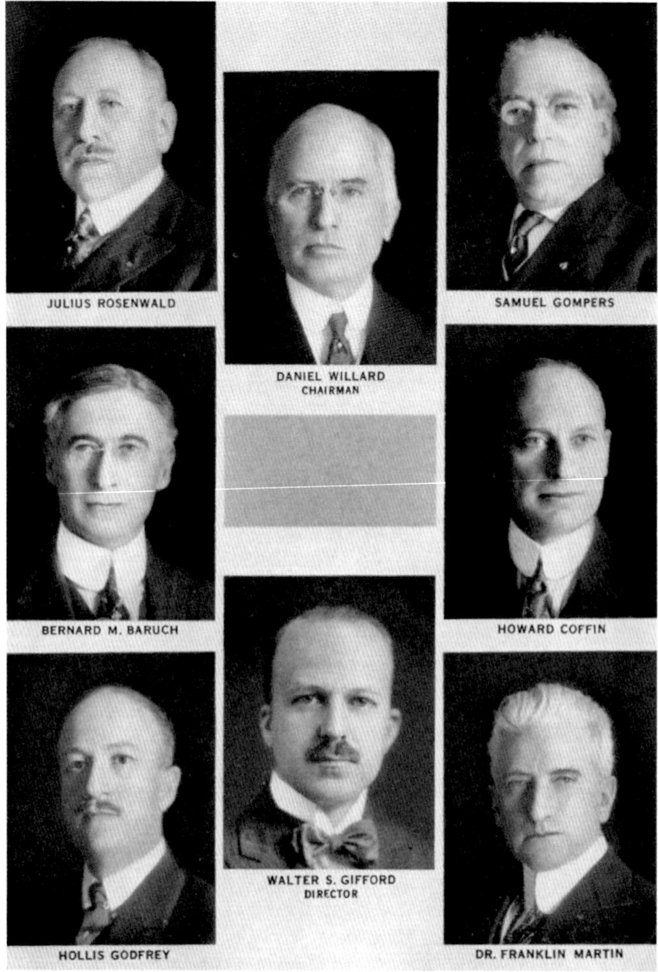

13.2. Members of the Advisory Commission of the Council of National Defense.

tin's protestations, Simpson succeeded in having President Woodrow Wilson appoint Martin to the Advisory Commission. As it turned out, Dr. Simpson's instincts were correct. Martin was a disciplined, highly organized, decisive leader and an excellent administator; he was an ideal choice to fill the position. Also appointed to the Commission were a railroad president (Daniel Willard), an engineer (Hollis Godfrey), a financier (Bernard Baruch), two businessmen (Julius Rosenwald and Howard Coffin), and a labor organizer

(Samuel Gompers) (Figure 13.2). Walter S. Gifford was appointed as Director of the Advisory Commission.[5] In President Wilson's words,

> The organization of the Council likewise opens up a new and direct channel of communication and co-operation between business and scientific men and all departments of the Government, and it is hoped that it will, in addition, become a rallying point for civic bodies working for the national defense.[6]

Martin's sense of pride at having been appointed to the Advisory Commission was now replaced with a growing sense of responsibility:

> The appointment was a command, and was so interpreted by each one of the seven men who were peremptorily summoned from positions of importance in private life to serve their Government, without remuneration, as members of the Advisory Commission.[6]

Martin Supports the Idea of Individual U.S. Hospitals Organizing American Base Hospitals for Military Service

Soon after his appointment to the Advisory Commission, Martin began meeting with Colonel Jefferson Kean, Director-General of Military Relief for the American National Red Cross, who was organizing base hospitals for military service. Dr. George W. Crile, of Lakeside Hospital and professor of surgery at Western Reserve University, Cleveland, had proposed that American base hospitals be organized around the personnel from a single U. S. hospital to avoid the strife and discord that might occur if individuals from multiple institutions were brought together to form a single base hospital.

Dr. Crile outlined in detail the logistics necessary to establish and run such a base hospital. He believed that regular Army officers should be responsible for hospital construction and administration, which would allow the physicians to devote their time to patient care. Colonel Kean championed this concept and convinced Martin of its utility. After a discussion with the Army Surgeon General, Martin reviewed in detail Dr. Crile's proposal for a 500-bed base hospital organized around a single U. S. hospital unit. As was the usual with Martin, once he was convinced of the correctness of a solution, he moved forward aggressively. Arrangements were made with the assistance of the Secretary of War to have Dr. Crile mobilize his Lakeside Hospital unit and place it on display at the Clinical Congress of the American College of Surgeons in Philadelphia in October 1916. On demonstration was a 500-bed base hospital along with physicians, surgeons, enlisted men, and nurses.[7] During the war, 129 U.S. base hospitals were organized similarly to the one Crile described and operated in either France or England. Six of these U.S. base hospital units were set up in Europe before any other military organizations from the United States arrived: Crile's Lakeside Hospital unit, Dr. Harvey Cushing's Harvard University unit, Dr. George E. Brewer's Presbyterian Hospital of New York City unit, Dr. Frederic A. Besley's Northwestern University unit, Dr. Richard H. Harte's Pennsylvania Hospital unit, and Dr. Fred T. Murphy's Washington University of St. Louis unit.[8]

Preliminary Organization of the Advisory Commission and the Council of National Defense

Martin and other members of the Advisory Commission were invited to Washington on December 6, 1916, for the initial organizational meeting of the Commission. Looking back, it is obvious that none of them realized the nature of the task they were expected to accomplish. Martin had a large surgical practice that he expected to return to after a short time in Washington. It did not cross his mind that he would never return to the practice of surgery.

On the evening before the first official meeting of the Advisory Commission, a dinner was arranged so that the members of the Commission could get better acquainted. They came away impressed with the President's selection of individuals for the Commission, especially with the labor leader Samuel Gompers.[9] The following day the seven members of the Advisory Commission had their introductory meeting with the six cabinet members comprising the Council of National Defense: Secretary of War Newton Diehl Baker, Secretary of the Navy Josephus Daniels, Secretary of the Interior Franklin K. Lane, Secretary of Agriculture David F. Houston, Secretary of Commerce William C. Redfield, and Secretary of Labor William B. Wilson (Figure 13.3). This meeting was followed by an official meeting with President Wilson at

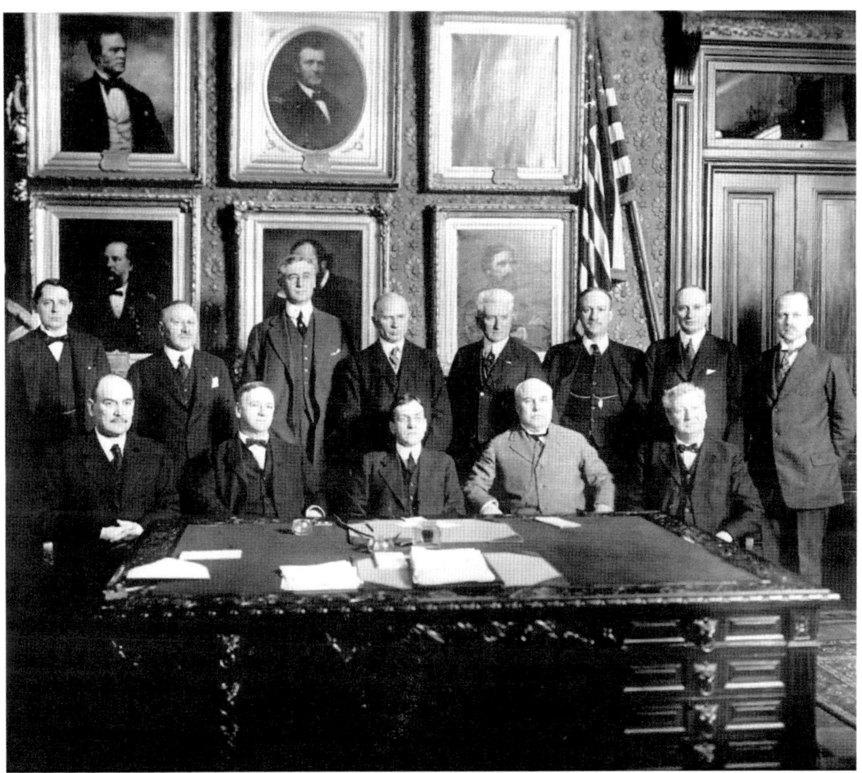

13.3. Members of the Council of National Defense and the Advisory Commission. Seated, from left: David F. Houston, Josephus Daniels, Newton D. Baker (Chairman), Franklin K. Lane, and William B. Wilson. Standing, from left: Grosvenor Clarkson (Secretary), Julius Rosenwald, Bernard Baruch, Daniel Willard, Franklin H. Martin, Hollis Godfrey, Howard Coffin, and Walter Gifford.

which he outlined what he anticipated the group would accomplish. This was followed by the first formal meeting of the Advisory Commission, at which a plan of organization was agreed upon, and Hollis Godfrey was appointed chairman.[10]

During multiple meetings of both the Council and Commission the following week, it became obvious to everyone that there was much that needed to be accomplished to prepare the United States for entry into the war. As they participated in their daily discussions, the members of the Advisory Commission began to comprehend the magnitude of the task at hand, and this realization united them. Martin believed that, as advisors, the members of the Advisory Commission were not bound by traditional government procedures and could use shortcuts to circumvent the hierarchical government structure. In their positions as leaders of large, nongovernment organizations they were accustomed to acting independently and could use that ability to circumvent the rules and regulations of the bureaucratic government departments with which they were now expected to work. This direct action obviously appealed to Martin because it was his preferred style of management and one at which he was very adept. At the same time, they were no longer autonomous individuals managing their private organizations, but instead were significant participants in a large government machine; they needed to discipline themselves and follow regulations as appropriate. It became obvious that the Advisory Commission members could enlist the assistance of experts in the business and professional community, thereby expanding the pool of available expertise to supplement the efforts of overworked government departments.[11]

After the early meetings of the Council of National Defense in December 1916, Martin described the activities of the Advisory Commission,

> ...we were carefully observing, making our notes, obtaining information, thinking out our obligations, and segregating our individual responsibilities, so that when we finally did advise action we would do it judiciously and effectively.[12]

From his previous behavior as an organizational administrator and leader, it is obvious that Martin would not tolerate rigidly following the rules and regulations of the U.S. government and the military services, especially when seeking approval for a new program. In other words, he wouldn't settle for starting at the bottom of the chain of command and working his way through the ranks to gain approval. Instead, he would prefer to go directly to the ultimate decision-maker, even if that meant going directly to President Wilson—which he did on occasion.[12]

At the early meetings of the Council and Commission, members expressed both anxiety and curiosity about the war efforts. Secretary of War Baker, Secretary of the Navy Daniels, Secretary of Labor Wilson, one member of the Advisory Commission, Mr. Gompers, and the President all were pacifists, but were still involved in the country's war preparations. Despite being pacifists, the three Cabinet Secretaries expressed the belief that increased preparedness would discourage the nation's enemies, and if the efforts were unsuccessful in discouraging them, the U.S. would be prepared to repel their aggression. Although Martin was not a pacifist, he had respect for the convictions of these men and the strength of their character in the face of the task at hand.[13]

Between meetings Martin and Dr. Simpson consulted frequently with the Surgeons General of the Army, Navy, and Public Health Service and Colonel Kean of the Red Cross. Simpson and Martin initially perceived a lack of collaboration between these groups, which would undoubtedly lead to ineffective administration of the distribution of medical care during war. Martin's keen observations of the interrelationship between these departments would serve him well during his tenure in Washington.[14]

OBTAINS APPROVAL FOR THE COMMITTEE OF AMERICAN PHYSICIANS FOR MEDICAL PREPAREDNESS TO BE A UNIT OF THE COUNCIL OF NATIONAL DEFENSE

Since its organization in April 1916, the Committee of American Physicians for Medical Preparedness had been surveying the country's medical resources and already had assisted in enrolling medical personnel into the Medical Reserve Corps, organizing Red Cross base hospitals, and acquiring and storing medical and surgical supplies. Such activities were acknowledged to be models for the future work of the Advisory Commission. In view of the group's effective work, Martin requested that the Committee of American Physicians for Medical Preparedness be incorporated into the Advisory Commission and be made a unit in the Medical Section of the Council of National Defense. His motion, his first since joining the Commission, was enthusiastically received and promptly adopted by the Council.[15] This is yet another example of Martin's particular ability to identify a problem that others might not perceive, design a solution for that problem, and expeditiously carry it through to its solution on his own initiative. During his time on the Advisory Commission, he would act similarly on numerous occasions.

Organizes a Meeting of Medical School Deans to Begin Preparing for War

With authorization from the Council and Advisory Commission, Martin invited the deans of all accredited U.S. medical schools to a January 6, 1917, conference in Washington. Ninety-five percent of the medical schools sent representatives. In his opening remarks, Martin informed the deans that the Army and Navy needed 5,000 new reserve medical officers and that the spring's 4,000 medical school graduates would be excellent candidates. Colonel William H. Arthur presented a special curriculum designed to prepare senior medical students to be Army medical officers.

After this presentation, the medical school deans passed a resolution directing the Secretary of War to supply each medical school with an instructor in military medicine and sanitation within four weeks and pledged to make this curriculum mandatory. The Council of National Defense later approved and authorized the resolution. With this ingenious plan, Martin had succeeded in assuring that all medical students graduating that year and in subsequent years would receive appropriate training for military service and be prepared to assist in the war effort. The Surgeons General of the Army, Navy, and Public Health Service were pleased by the response of the medical school deans. Martin also was encouraged by the deans' sympathetic response, and he made initial plans for a campaign to recruit practicing physicians into the Medical Corps.[16]

Martin Insists on Thorough Record-Keeping

After the first few weeks of meetings, Martin became dissatisfied with the poor documentation of the meetings of the Council of National Defense and Advisory Commission and moved that complete minutes of all committee meetings be recorded. These minutes would leave a more complete record for future historical review. In addition, at the next meeting of the Advisory Commission he made a motion, which was adopted unanimously, that all meetings be conducted under parliamentary rules to ensure that every issue received proper discussion. Until this rule was adopted, subjects of great importance that should have received a thorough Advisory Commission discussion before being presented to the Council often were glossed over, whereas less significant issues were discussed at length.[17] Martin, a highly organized administrator, had the insight to see the need for these changes.

STANDARDIZATION OF SURGICAL INSTRUMENTS, SURGICAL DRESSINGS, AND PHARMACEUTICALS

Martin had become aware that civilian committees of several organizations were attempting to standardize surgical instruments, surgical dressings, and medical pharmaceuticals. He proposed, and it was accepted, that these committees be invited to Washington for a joint meeting with the Medical Section of the Council, the Surgeons General of the Army and Navy, and the Medical Director of the Red Cross. It also was agreed that the War Department furnish storage facilities for medical supplies that were being collected by private organizations—a wonderful demonstration of how Martin always took a global approach to a problem, evaluating all its aspects and addressing each detail directly, analagous to the way he handled learning how the complex machinery in his uncle's flour mill functioned.[18]

DIVISION OF THE ADVISORY COMMISSION INTO COMMITTEES

Because of issues like those described previously, which would benefit from additional coordination and preparation before presentation to the Advisory Commission, it was proposed and adopted that the Commission be divided into committees, with members of the commission serving as chairs. Martin's Medicine Committee included general sanitation. Each committee chair had the power to select members for his committee from both the government and private industry. With this change, the committees were expected to formulate a plan of action for any perceived problem or need before it was presented to the Advisory Commission. Proposals approved by the Commission were then forwarded to the Council of National Defense for consideration. In addition, the Council would furnish the Commission with a list of materials and services that likely would affect the national defense and welfare of the country in time of war. The process would include a series of conferences with representatives of appropriate trades, businesses, and professions to address specific problems.

Martin was especially interested in these developments because his work to date had proceeded along a similar line of action. For instance, before he approached medical school deans about preparing senior medical students for service in the military, he first received approval from the Council and Commission. Because of the complex nature of many of the issues, Martin had created an Executive Committee of the Medical Committee of the Advisory Council, which discussed plans in detail; only when the plans were approved by the Executive Committee were they forwarded to the Advisory Commission. This structure enabled the medical committee to aid the government and the military. Because of this effective approach, the services of the Medical Committee in designing action plans were in constant demand.[19]

Authorization by the Council of National Defense to Enlarge the Medical Committee

With the restructuring of the Advisory Commission by creating committees under the chairmanship of the seven commissioners, and because of the increased demand for the Medical Committee's services, Martin sought and received permission from the Council of National Defense to greatly enlarge his committee, which he then called the General Medical Board.[20] In the process, he created 30 separate committees and subcommittees populated with experts from within and outside of government, all working to address specific issues that would affect the nation in the event of war. All the committee and subcommittee members were selected by Martin and he knew that he could depend on them to make appropriate and well-conceived decisions.[21]

The General Medical Board was authorized by the Council of National Defense to be a cooperating agency between the medical officers enrolled from civilian life and the regular Army, Navy, and Public Health Service medical departments. At the Board's initial meeting on April 9, 1917, Martin assured the Surgeons General on the board that this truly would be a cooperating body and that working together would allow them to comprehend more thoroughly the medical problems of war. Martin was concerned that the barrier of the chain of command could hamper effective communications between government departments and the military, as well as between the

General Medical Board civilians and government departments. In the end, Martin succeeded in simplifying communications between these groups and, in the process, created a more businesslike atmosphere within and outside of government for everyone involved. The resulting open communications helped to avoid duplicative efforts and proposals that might be embarrassing to a branch of the military. Most importantly, it meant that proposals brought forward to the Council of National Defense had already been thoroughly discussed and approved by the General Medical Board and its Executive Committee. As noted previously, Martin believed that this style of communication within an organization was the most expeditious way to obtain approval for proposals at the highest level. Of course, on many occasions Martin already had a clear vision of the most appropriate solution for a problem and would simply use these well-designed lines of communication to obtain approval for a solution he had already outlined.

The General Medical Board convened on Sunday mornings and were always well attended. Medical representatives of the Allied governments, U.S. government leaders, international leaders, and members of the medical, surgical, dental, and nursing professions often were invited to attend. Under Martin's guidance, everyone was encouraged to contribute suggestions and ideas to the group discussions. Drs. William and Charles Mayo, Dr. Victor Vaughan of Ann Arbor, Dr. William Welsh of Baltimore, Dr. Frederic A. Besley of Chicago, and Dr. George W. Crile of Cleveland were frequent attendees.[22]

Identified the Importance of Controlling the Food Supply during War

Although the Commission acknowledged that price-fixing as it related to control of the wartime food supply was an important issue, after a half-day's discussion the group was unable to formulate an effective plan to deal with the problem. Price fixing's effect on the availability of adequate quantities of proper food not only affected the health of military personnel, but also that of the civilian population; so, this problem required expeditious action. Price fixing also affected the supply of grain, cotton, wool, and other raw materials. It occurred to Martin that control of the food supply for a nation at war was basically a health problem and, therefore, should be the responsibility of the Committee on Medicine and Sanitation.[23]

At the next Advisory Commission meeting, Martin proposed placing the regulation of the price and conservation of foods under the control of an administrative board that would report to the Council of National Defense and the President. Martin suggested Mr. Herbert Hoover as chair of the proposed administrative board because of his administrative acumen. At the next meeting of the Council, the proposal passed and was immediately enacted by the President.[24]

Interestingly, the Secretary of Agriculture suggested that his department should supervise the regulation of food prices and conservation and that they had already discussed a similar plan. Martin answered that it mattered little who had been discussing a solution, but it was imperative that a concrete program be outlined and brought forward—which he had done.[25] As Martin had experienced many times in the past, when others wavered, he acted. It was his evaluation that, over time, the entire Advisory Commission used his methods when developing a plan of action. To quote Martin, "All these and a multitude of other questions, depending upon varying circumstances and difficulties, were before us for solution. There was no time for long and tedious discussions; there could be no procrastination in decision."[26]

Program Controlling the Consumption of Alcohol by and the Exposure to Venereal Disease of Military Personnel

Martin scheduled a conference for April 15–16, 1917, to discuss the problem of venereal disease in the military and the principal contributing factor to its occurrence: excessive use of alcoholic beverages. The leading professional and lay authorities on venereal disease and alcohol use attended the conference, which was directed by the Committee on Hygiene and Sanitation of the General Medical Board and its Subcommittees on Venereal Disease and Alcohol Control.

The conference report on venereal disease included the following resolutions:

- That the Departments of War and Navy officially recognize that sexual continence [abstaining from sexual activity] is compatible with health and that it is the best prevention of venereal infections.

- That the Departments of War and Navy take steps toward the prevention of venereal infections through exclusion of prostitutes within an effective zone surrounding all places under their control, and by the provision of suitable recreational facilities, the control of the use of alcoholic drinks, and other effective measures.

- That the said Departments adopt a plan for centralized control of venereal infections through special divisions of their medical services.[27]

The main issues identified were the importance of alcohol use as a factor in the spread of venereal diseases, the disabling effects of these diseases on military personnel during and after their service, and the negative impact on the food supply of the enormous quantities of food materials used to manufacture alcoholic beverages.

The President, Cabinet officers, and members of the Advisory Commission received numerous telegrams and letters in opposition to the General Medical Board's plan. Nonetheless, President Wilson and the Secretary of War continued to express their approval of the plan. The resolutions on venereal disease and the use of alcoholic beverages were adopted with minimal changes. This regulation had a far-reaching effect on the military and the country. It was Martin's belief that the parents of young men eligible to serve in the military welcomed this regulation controlling the use of alcoholic beverages. The impact on society was significant, and in Martin's mind it led to an increase in the number of people supporting Prohibition. Soon this regulation, which originally only applied to soldiers in camps, was extended to include any soldier in uniform, wherever he might be.[27]

Martin prepared a press statement concerning the control of venereal diseases and the regulation of the use of alcohol in the Army and Navy that was approved after modification by the Council of National Defense:

> Zones about the military commands will...be created and conditions in these zones will be guarded by military measures so as to prevent the spread of venereal diseases. The two military arms of the Government officially recognize that continence [abstaining from sexual activity] is compatible with health.

> The Council also recommends, as a further solution to the problem, that all military commands be provided with good facilities for the recreation of the troops. It urges that all suitable athletics be encouraged.
>
> The use of alcoholic beverages on the part of soldiers and sailors in military commands has long been under military control. But the creation now of these military zones will in effect extend such control over the troops when they are off duty out of the commands....[28]

To help carry out the provision for recreation facilities, the Council appointed the Fosdick Commission on Training Camp Activities, chaired by Raymond B. Fosdick. In a broad sense, the Fosdick Commission organized and unified these activities at all military commands.[29]

By all accounts, this program was successful, enough so that, with Martin's backing, the Committee on Hygiene and Sanitation and its Subcommittee on Alcohol Control recommended that the same regulations addressing the consumption of alcoholic beverages by troops stationed at military commands in the U.S. be enforced when the troops were in Europe. The committee also wanted the President to request the British and French governments to enforce this program for American troops. The request was not well accepted by the French and British armies but was solidly supported by General John Pershing, Commander-in-Chief of the American Expeditionary Forces in Europe. He had experience with the effects of venereal disease on soldiers; it rendered them inefficient as soldiers and made them an encumbrance to their command. Pershing carried the regulation further by banning the acceptance of alcoholic beverages as gifts.[30]

This policy had an amazing impact. In past wars, a venereal disease infection rate of 25 percent was considered normal, and the profound effects of these diseases continued when soldiers returned home. In an era when minimal effective treatment was available, venereal disease could result in deformity, prolonged misery, and even death. With this new policy, fewer than 1 percent of soldiers had venereal disease at the time of discharge after World War I.[31] Martin identified and solved this problem in the face of overwhelming odds against such a policy being approved.

Martin believed that the impact of the prohibition of alcohol consumption by American troops was more profound than was seen initially. He observed,

> While I am sure the authors of the resolutions did not realize what the consequence might be, nor contemplate any action beyond the control of venereal diseases, the effect was dynamic. Every father and mother of the 5,000,000 civilian boys who were eligible as volunteers or draftees, whether or not the parents themselves had prohibitionary tendencies, welcomed this regulation that would control the use of alcoholic beverages in camps and overseas.... This measure profoundly influenced the minds of the civilian population of the Nation. Was there ever a more fertile soil or a more promising atmosphere in which the propagandist for temperance could ply his work? The momentum developed by this wartime measure of the medical profession was a firm foundation for the peacetime eighteenth amendment.[32]

BRITISH REQUEST FOR DOCTORS

At a reception for the Right Honorable Arthur J. Balfour of Great Britain, Mr. Balfour approached Martin and requested that the United States send physicians both to the front, where they were desperately needed, and to Great Britain, where they would help care for the civilian population. Balfour requested 1,000 physicians; in view of the tremendous need, Martin offered to send 2,000. He agreed to a meeting the following day with Mr. Balfour's military aide, and at that time formally agreed to send 1,000 physicians. He had made this offer without prior approval from the Secretary of War, Newton D. Baker. But he went immediately to Mr. Baker's office to obtain approval—which was given, despite some irritation on Baker's part. If a similar request had been made by Mr. Balfour to any other member of the Advisory Commission, they likely would have referred the request to the Commission and probably the Council, and only then sought approval from Secretary Baker. But Martin knew that the United States must support Great Britain, so he did what he believed was right. In his mind, under such circumstances, the chain of command was something that had to be circumvented.[33]

Recruiting Doctors for the Medical Reserve Corps

One of Martin's major assignments as the medical member of the Advisory Commission was the recruitment of physicians for the Medical Reserve Corps, a duty he performed with distinction. His first experiences with persuading physicians to enroll in the Corps was at a war rally at the 1917 American Medical Association annual meeting. When the invited guest speakers did not show, Martin was asked to speak. Although uneasy and speaking extemporaneously, he spoke for an hour. He gave an impassioned speech, beginning by asserting that the physicians and surgeons of the country had failed to rise to the call of duty. Besides the needs of the United States, Great Britain and France were begging for doctors, and Martin believed the United States should be sending at least 500 physicians a month.[34]

Although he was uncomfortable at the beginning of his speech that night, by the end he was invigorated and felt he had made a significant impression on his audience. Because of this experience, he organized a series of patriotic meetings across the country to encourage physician enrollment in the Medical Reserve Corps. The first three of these meetings were scheduled for Chicago, Minneapolis, and Rochester, MN. The reason these efforts were so vitally important was that, at the beginning of the war, the Army had slightly fewer than 500 of the 30,000 physicians necessary to treat an army of 5 million men.

This maldistribution of medical professionals placed a tremendous responsibility on Martin and his committee, because although medical personnel recruitment was their primary undertaking, they needed to address many other challenges.[35] These tasks included ensuring the health of the troops, conserving resources, rehabilitating the wounded, and addressing venereal disease. For the remainder of the war, Martin crisscrossed the country giving speeches encouraging physicians to enroll in the Medical Reserve Corps. This effort was time-consuming but effective and offered Martin the opportunity to attend the meetings of many national, state, and local medical societies. On one tour of the upper and lower Midwest, he gave talks at 10 meetings and all met with excellent response.[36]

INTERESTING COMPLAINT

Dr. Charles Mayo called Martin to his Washington office July 26, 1918, to discuss a disturbing talk he'd had with the Assistant Secretary of War, Frederick Keppel, who had suggested that Martin might be dismissed from the Advisory Council because he had antagonized someone from a medical-political group. Martin was unperturbed and stated that in the performance of his work he was responsible only to the President of the United States, and that he was attempting to do his job to the best of his ability.[37] This is the answer you would expect from a man who always kept in mind whom he was serving, especially when he was convinced that he had made an appropriate decision. Under such conditions, the fact that other individuals disagreed with his plan was secondary.

INCREASING THE RANK FOR MEDICAL OFFICERS

Early in the war, the highest rank attainable for medical officers was colonel in the regular Army Medical Corps and major in the Medical Reserve Corps. Consequently, many highly qualified American physicians held the rank of major, whereas their British and French physician counterparts held the rank of colonel and even general—even though they were performing the same professional duties. This difference in rank was at times humiliating to American physicians, who felt inferior to the British and French medical officers.

At a meeting on June 25, 1917, the General Medical Board approved a bill providing for increased rank for medical officers. The bill was presented with amendments in both Houses of Congress, with the support of President Wilson and the Secretary of War. The bill met with opposition and initially failed to achieve passage. Martin, with the aid of the General Medical Board, contacted state and county medical committees throughout the United States, requesting that they lobby their senators and representatives about the issue. Despite this effort, it appeared that the bill would be defeated. Martin appealed again to the President. With President Wilson's support, the bill passed in July 1918. The bill gave physicians the ranks from lieutenant to major general—the same ranks afforded to British and French medical officers.[38]

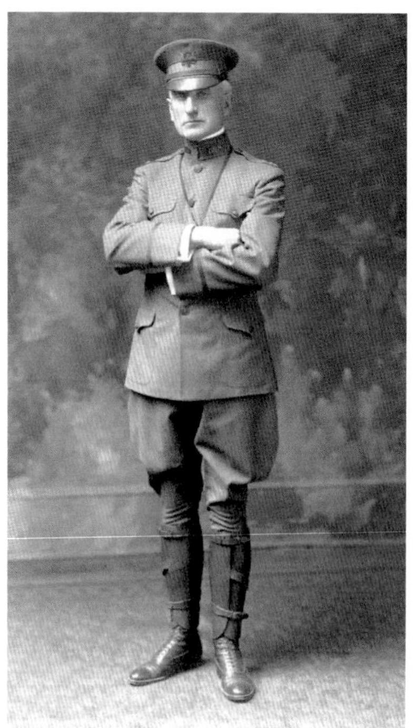

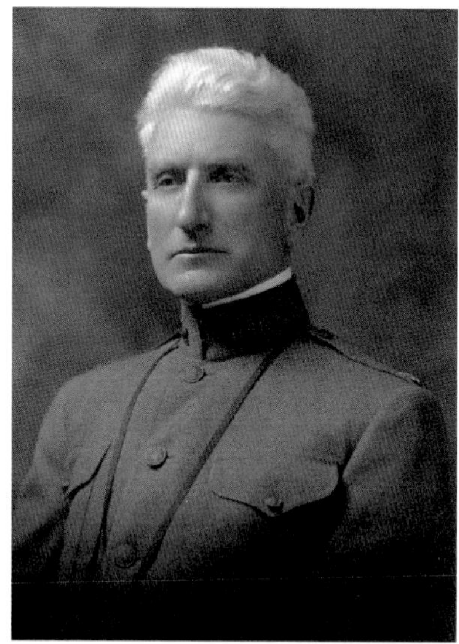

13.4. Martin in his Army uniform.

Creation of the Volunteer Medical Service Corps

Many physicians who had been rejected for active duty in the Medical Reserve Corps because of physical and medical limitations, for being past the age limit, or because they were needed for responsibilities at home, still wanted to help with the war effort. Many of them were fit, capable, and acceptable for home duty or administrative duty at the front but would need an appointment and an insignia or uniform to establish their authority. Martin discussed this idea with President Wilson, the Secretary of War, the Surgeons General, his own staff, and members of his Executive Committee. Surgeon General William C. Gorgas suggested a Volunteer Medical Service Corps. At a special meeting January 31, 1918, the Council of National Defense created the Corps and authorized an insignia. President Wilson approved the plan. Dr. Edward P. Davis of Philadelphia was named president of the Central Governing Board of the new Corps and appointed several eminent physicians to the board. He established state committees to oversee the affairs of the Corps. Once the existence of the Corps was announced, it received 100,000 membership applications.

Soon after the Corps creation, the U.S. Public Health Service requested assistance in combating the 1918 influenza epidemic on the East Coast. All segments of the population were succumbing to the epidemic, and physicians were desperately needed. Physicians who practiced in the affected area were working day and night, and every hospital was being taxed to its limit. The Public Health Service asked the Volunteer Medical Service Corps to send 500 physicians to Massachusetts within 24 hours to help control the epidemic. In his absence, Dr. Martin's secretary, Florence Donnelly—as Martin would have done—agreed that she would immediately send the names of 500 physicians. Within 24 hours, the Public Health Service received the names of 700 physicians, and eventually 1,200 names came in.

At its strongest, the Volunteer Medical Service Corps had 72,219 physician members. In creating the Corps, Martin had again risen to the occasion—something that the Surgeons General alone were ill-prepared to have accomplished.[39]

SUMMARY OF WAR YEARS

Looking back, there is little doubt that Martin was the best choice to represent the medical profession on the Advisory Commission of the Council of National Defense (Figure 13.4). His organizational abilities, his talent for designing thorough solutions for complex problems, his effectiveness in forging ahead when others might waver, and his untiring energy when fighting for a cause he believed in were attributes that served him well in this position. In my mind, few other prominent physicians, except for Dr. Frank Simpson, could have performed at the level that he did.

Of Martin's service during World War I Admiral Cary T. Grayson said:

> ...he demonstrated to an unusual degree the rare gifts of administrative genius and vision.[40]

> Franklin Martin was above all a good soldier. He was brave; he was fearless; he would not recognize defeat, and once he had determined on a course, his generalship,

> untiring energy, and fighting force could be depended upon to see him through to a successful conclusion.[41]

What a wonderful testimonial to Martin's leadership abilities, especially coming from a Navy Rear Admiral.

References

1. Martin, F. H. (1933). *The Joy of Living: An Autobiography*, vol. 2 (pp. 1-29). New York, NY: Doubleday, Doran & Co.
2. Sped through lines as German royalty: Flag on auto of Chicago surgeon enabled him to go from Holland to Munich and back. (1914, August 22). *New York Times*, p. 3.
3. Nahrwold, D. L. (2018). The rescue of Miss Inez Stone. *Bull Am Coll Surg*, 103(7), 62-63.
4. Martin, F. H. (1933). *The Joy of Living: An Autobiography*, vol. 2 (pp. 38-42). New York, NY: Doubleday, Doran & Co.
5. Ibid., pp. 43-48.
6. Ibid., pp. 48-51.
7. Ibid., pp. 53-57.
8. Ibid., pp. 173-175.
9. Ibid., pp. 60-63.
10. Ibid., pp. 64-67.
11. Ibid., pp. 67-72.
12. Ibid., p. 79.
13. Ibid., pp. 74-76.
14. Ibid., pp. 76-77.
15. Ibid., pp. 72-73.
16. Ibid., pp. 79-82.
17. Ibid., pp. 83-84.
18. Ibid., pp. 87-88.
19. Ibid., pp. 90-92.
20. Ibid., pp. 116-117.
21. Ibid., pp. 118 and 473-487.
22. Ibid., pp. 130-135.
23. Ibid., p. 118.

24. Ibid., pp. 119-120.
25. Ibid., p. 120.
26. Ibid., p. 127.
27. Ibid., pp. 138-144.
28. Ibid., p. 145.
29. Ibid., pp. 338-339.
30. Ibid., pp. 339-341.
31. Baker, D. B. Foreword. In: Martin, F. H. (1933). *The Joy of Living: An Autobiography,* vol. 2 (p. xiii). New York, NY: Doubleday, Doran & Co.
32. Martin, F. H. (1933). *The Joy of Living: An Autobiography,* vol. 2 (p. 144). New York, NY: Doubleday, Doran & Co.
33. Ibid., pp. 155-161.
34. Ibid., pp. 180-186.
35. Ibid., pp. 245-246.
36. Ibid., pp. 323-335.
37. Ibid., p. 345.
38. Ibid., pp. 346-350.
39. Ibid., pp. 377-385.
40. Grayson, C. T. (1935). Franklin H. Martin and the Great War. *Bull Am Coll Surg,* 20(2), 53.
41. Ibid., p. 55.

Chapter 14

Advancing the College— 1917 to 1935

oon moved ov… those ~~[illegible]~~ thought t
that the Corliss Sunday had Every bo
Jessins on the big head. … i
claim on the big bend. Volunteers
the raising on Saturday. Volunteers
~~[illegible]~~ were busy from all the neig
the week, felling trees, and hewing ~~the~~ addition
the shop for the new house. Early
g of Saturday a dozen or more s
nd boys were on hand to construc
house. A cellar had been dug in th
~~[illegible]~~ ready to be encased with ston
…in logs had been sunk in tren
ached a bed of solid clay beneath th
il, lumber had been brought from
aw mill and a fine lot of dry c
been contributed by generous neighbors
er ~~[illegible]~~ ready to compete with Su
Sunday oxen that had been brou
neighbors.

Jim Inslee by common cons
of the game
foreman for the day. No time was
all directions came the great logs
iron chains about their necks a
… of the faithful oxen

MARTIN APPOINTED FULL-TIME SECRETARY-GENERAL OF THE ACS IN OCTOBER 1917

At the October 1917 American College of Surgeons (ACS) Clinical Congress, the Regents decided to offer Dr. Martin a full-time position as chief administrative officer, with the title of Secretary-General. Unlike in the past, when he had been the General Secretary of the ACS and declined remuneration for his services, with this appointment he was to receive a full-time salary. Drs. William Mayo, George W. Crile, and Edward Martin came to Martin's bedside at the Congress Hotel, where he was recovering from pneumonia, to report this decision. Martin had planned to return to his large, lucrative surgical practice in Chicago after the war, and accepting this position would make returning to practice impossible. He asked that the three men not force him to make such an important decision while he was ill. They agreed, saying they would return the following morning for his final decision. Upon their return, and in spite of his misgivings, he heeded his wife's advice and accepted the position, stating, "These three of my best friends I am now convinced were primarily interested in the College, and I have never regretted my final yielding to their insistent plan."[1]

Before Martin accepted the Secretary-General position, his surgical practice and more recently his membership in the Advisory Commission of the Council of National Defense had not allowed him to take on full management of the College. In 1915, the College had hired John G. Bowman as Director, and he became actively immersed in managing the College. Martin's part-time assignment as General Secretary of the College had offered minimal opportunities to clash with Bowman, but the new arrangement certainly created the potential for conflict. To avoid such a possibility, Bowman and Martin agreed to revising the bylaws of the College to create two chief executive officer positions. As Secretary-General, Martin would be the chief executive and would supervise the general activities and business affairs of the College.

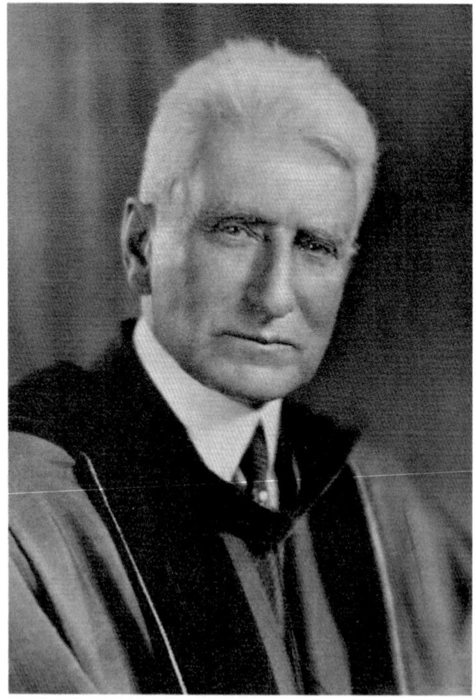

14.1. Martin circa 1930.

As Director, Bowman would oversee all educational activities, including admission to Fellowship, the hospital standardization program, and other related issues.

Although there were no obvious major disagreements between the two men, they had a trying, and at times difficult, relationship. Likely due in part to the awkwardness of having two chief executive officers, Bowman decided to leave the College in late 1920 to become Chancellor of the University of Pittsburgh. Eventually Judge Harold Stephens accepted the position of Director on a trial basis, but after five months he declined the full-time position. Before he left, Stephens made several recommendations to the Regents, the most important being that the College should have only a single chief executive officer. He said that having divided governance was "foreign to the fundamental principles of executive organization." The Board of Regents agreed, and in 1922 made Martin the College's sole chief executive officer, with supervision of all activities and business affairs and with the title Director-General.

This change in the bylaws gave Martin full control of the ACS under the direction of the Board of Regents (Figure 14.1).[2]

IMPORTANT PROGRAMS ESTABLISHED OR CHAMPIONED BY MARTIN

Under Martin's leadership the College developed many new programs and became a multifaceted organization. In Martin's view,

> The purposes of the American College of Surgeons are concerned directly with matters of character and of training, with the betterment of hospitals and of the teaching facilities of medical schools, with practical research, with laws which relate to medical practice and privilege, and with an unselfish protection of the public from incompetent service. The College aims to include within its Fellowship those surgeons who are competent in the art and technique of surgery.[3]

Under Martin's management the hospital standardization program continued to be a principal mission of the College and became a major expense. The program's impact continued to grow, as demonstrated by the fact that the hospital approval rate grew from an initial rate of less than 15 percent to 69 percent by 1929. This growth occurred even though the standards remained the same. Furthermore, hospital length of stay and mortality rates had been reduced. This successful program stayed under the direction of the ACS until the Joint Commission on Accreditation of Hospitals began managing the program in 1952. There is little doubt that without the guidance and unwavering support of Martin and the work of the hospital standardization program the quality of U.S. and Canadian hospitals would have stagnated or shown only minimal improvement for many years.[4]

Another successful program began in 1920 as a series of ACS state meetings, designed as a solution to the expense and time involved for surgeons to travel to and attend the Clinical Congress. In a little more than a year, 38 meetings were held throughout the U.S. and Canada. Although a large percentage of Fellows of the College attended the state meetings, such a schedule was unsustainable. So, Martin changed the format to one of sectional meetings involving multiple states and provinces, with a format like that of the Clinical Congress. During the sectional meetings, the College hosted presentations on the hospital standardization program, addresses by nationally prominent surgeons, and public meetings on medical topics for local laypeople. The public meetings were especially well attended, and the College's use of public relations methods for promotion contributed to their success. The sectional meetings continued for more than 50 years until they were phased out in 1973 because of decreasing attendance.[5]

In 1921 the Bone Sarcoma Registry was established to accumulate information about patients with this rare cancer, because no single surgeon or institution could collect enough cases to study and improve the diagnosis and treatment of the disease. Surgeons, pathologists, and radiologists reviewed the cases submitted to the registry. Because of this effort, a standardized nomenclature for bone sarcoma was developed, making it feasible to evaluate treatment outcomes. This successful program served as a model for future registries.[6]

In 1922 the College established a Committee on Fractures to develop fundamental, standard principles for the care and treatment of patients with fractures. The committee's recommendations were distributed to physicians and surgeons and to hospitals and other institutions. In addition, the College adopted a new standard that required approved hospitals to have the equipment and facilities to treat fractures. In concert with the Committee on Fractures, in 1927 the College appointed a Board of Industrial Medicine and Traumatic Surgery with the goal of creating adequate, scientific, and ethical care of ill and injured workers. The board recommended minimum standards for physicians and surgeons working in industrial clinics.[7]

Dr. George W. Crile said of Martin's accomplishments as leader of the ACS,

> The American College of Surgeons has had far-reaching influence on hospital standards, on ethical standards, on the standards of surgical practice, and on medical education. It was the conception of Franklin Martin that the College of Surgeons should be an active organization with comprehensive field activities covering the United States and Canada so completely that every hospital, whether in the metropolis or in remote places, should be served.... The machinery of these vast activities which spread all over the

continent and are carried on with vigor and judgment for the benefit of the public, is largely due to Franklin Martin.[8]

FOREIGN TRAVEL

In January 1920, as representatives of the College, Martin and William Mayo visited Panama, Peru, Chile, Argentina, and Uruguay to establish ties with South American surgeons. An equally successful visit was made in 1923 and expanded to include Columbia and Venezuela. Regrettably, some ACS members believed these trips deviated from the purpose of the College.

In 1924 Martin and William Mayo, independent of the College, traveled to Australia and New Zealand with the intention of making personal contact with surgeons in those countries. At the resulting meetings and conferences, the two men were asked to discuss the ACS and its hospital standardization program. As a follow-up, in 1926 the College's Associate Director of Hospital Activities, Dr. Malcolm MacEachern, traveled to Australia and New Zealand on behalf of the College to advise the countries regarding hospital standardization. Another outcome of the visits was that the Royal Australasian College of Surgeons was organized along lines that closely paralleled the ACS.[9]

CHALLENGES TO MARTIN'S LEADERSHIP

In the 1920s and 1930s, Martin faced significant challenges to his leadership of the College. In the 1920s, more than 6,000 surgeons were awarded Fellowship in the College, with a higher percentage coming from less urban and nonacademic environments. Surgeons from academic environments criticized the College leadership, contending that ACS admission standards were too low, and that Fellowship in the College was being devalued.

In 1924 two surgical groups, the Society of Clinical Surgery (SCS) and the Eclat Club (a group of surgeons who had served on the front lines during World War I), officially expressed dissatisfaction with the direction the leadership was taking the College. They recommended that the College reduce the number of new Fellows accepted by instituting more rigorous tests of character, training, and surgical acumen; they asserted that the ACS was allowing known fee splitters to become Fellows. Both

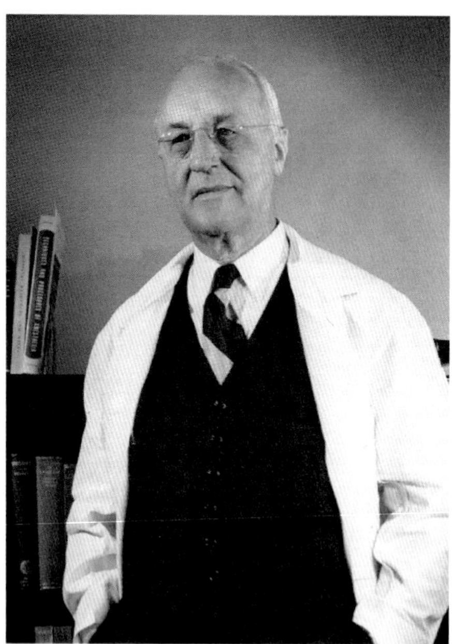

14.2. Dr. Evarts A. Graham, chair of surgery, Washington University in St. Louis, 1919 to 1951.

groups believed that the College's leaders were placing too little emphasis on clinical research. The Eclat Club wanted higher standards to be set for hospitals and wanted the College to issue annual financial statements. The Club also maintained that the Regents should assume more responsibility and gain more control over the direction of the College.[10]

The rising number of young, full-time academic surgeons—with Dr. Evarts A. Graham, chairman of surgery at Washington University, St. Louis, as their spokesman (Figure 14.2)—were unhappy with their lack of representation in the College management and believed that a small group of insiders controlled the College. On October 10, 1933, Dr. Graham presented his case to the Board of Regents. Most of his comments corresponded closely with the concerns members of the Eclat Club and the SCS expressed nine years earlier. The hierarchy of the College was divided on how to respond to Graham's presentation. Many of the Regents believed that an attempt at a compromise solution would be appropriate, but this did not occur, and the protesters remained alienated from the College.[11]

The Regents and Martin thought that changing the qualifications for membership in the College was unwise and that the present standards did not need to be made more stringent with the goal of decreasing the membership. Martin and the Regents believed that making membership available only to an elite group of surgeons, as practiced by the SCS and the Eclat Club, would benefit neither the medical profession nor patients. It was better to have more surgeons with an acceptable level of competence benefit from College membership and attendance at the annual Congress and the sectional meetings. Increasing surgical competence had always been Martin's goal, and to this day the College and patients have benefited from his stance in this matter.

Fee splitting always was and continued to be a contentious problem. (See a more detailed discussion of the practice later in this chapter.) Proving that a surgeon was splitting fees with his referring physicians could be very difficult and could result in defamation lawsuits. It was wise for the College to only disallow membership to surgeons who were openly and obviously involved in fee splitting. To have done otherwise could have been a public relations disaster and could have led to financial difficulties for the College.

The SCS and the Eclat Club were not necessarily aware that Martin, with the backing of the Regents, had considered their recommended changes but had rejected them as not being in the best interests of the College. Regrettably Martin took challenges to his leadership like this very personally and was frequently enraged by such encounters.[12]

Impact of Martin's Stroke on the ACS

In April 1930, at 73 years old, Martin had a left hemispheric cerebral infarction. As a consequence, he developed amnesia, aphasia, and right-sided hemiplegia. His recovery was slow, but by the end of July he had resumed some of his duties at the College. By October, he had no residual deficit that could be easily detected by anyone unaware of his stroke. Interestingly, the occurrence of the stroke and its aftereffects were not reported to the ACS membership and were omitted from his autobiography. By all appearances, the College functioned normally during his absence, and he was able to resume his duties as Director-General. Reading his autobiography and the observations of others, he seemed less robust and clear-thinking after his stroke.[13]

Impact of the Depression on the ACS and Martin's Response

In 1931, because of the Great Depression and a decrease in dues income, the College reduced its staff from 37 to 26. The remaining staff, including Martin, took 10 percent pay cuts. Martin's leadership style had earned him the respect and admiration of the College staff, and morale remained strong during the Depression.[14]

Health Insurance Issues and Disagreement with the AMA

The chief reason for the animosity between the College and the American Medical Association (AMA) was the AMA's determination to be the sole representative of American organized medicine, a privilege that Dr. Martin and the ACS were unwilling to grant. To have done so would have made the College subordinate to the AMA and left it unable to truly represent surgeons and surgery on national issues such as health insurance. If Martin had not, throughout his career, kept the College the strong advocate for surgeons that it was, surgeons would have been at the mercy of the AMA, which by design was not an advocate for surgeons' interests. The College would not be the robust organization it is today without Martin's leadership and steadfastness.[15]

In the 1920s, the cost of health care began to increase with the growth of hospitals, technology, and medical specialization. In 1932, the Milbank Foundation Committee on the Costs of Medical Care recommended that group practices provide medical services and that insurance coverage be made available to cover medical costs and lost wages, that there should be a greater emphasis on prevention and public health, that health care should be coordinated using community and state agencies, and that there should be improved education for all health care providers. The AMA condemned the report and its representatives on the committee issued a minority report justifying solo, fee-for-service practice and maintaining that it was the only acceptable model for health care delivery. The College, in part because of its involvement in the hospital standardization program, believed that hospitals faced financial problems that would be improved if patients had insurance coverage. The Depression and the resultant 25 percent unemployment rate increased the concerns about the cost of medical care. The inability of an increasing number of indigent patients to pay for medical care affected physician incomes and hospital finances. Hospital insurance programs and prepaid care programs began to appear. The AMA opposed all insurance programs and labeled them "socialized medicine," whereas the College displayed an interest in such programs.

At Martin's request, in March 1933, the Regents appointed a new committee, the Medical Service Board, to study how best to provide adequate medical services at a cost the public could afford. In the final report, the College endorsed voluntary prepayment plans for hospital and medical services for patients of moderate means. The Regents asserted that care for the indigent should be the obligation of the community and that physicians caring for the indigent should receive remuneration. The College's endorsement of prepayment for services once again put it in conflict with the AMA. As would be expected, the AMA passed a resolution claiming that the AMA had the sole right to speak for the American medical profession. The AMA trustees followed with a letter to the College Regents demanding an explanation for their actions. Martin was opposed to any meetings with the AMA about the subject and commented,

> They had invited us repeatedly and it has always been an insult. Why do we have to deal with them at all? ...I have had experience with these people. There is no help in them. Give them a lee-way, and that is all they want. Let us invite them and then you will be sorry; I will tell you that.[16]

Such a comment from Martin is unsurprising in view of his long history of conflict and antagonism with the AMA. When Martin felt secure in his beliefs, as he did with this issue, he would not allow another organization to control the College's actions.[16]

Martin's Relationship with Dr. Bevan and the AMA

Even before Martin's 1905 establishment of *Surgery, Gynecology & Obstetrics,* but certainly with its creation, his relationship with the AMA and specifically Dr. Arthur Dean Bevan, the first chair of the

AMA Council on Medical Education, became increasingly contentious and failed to improve during Martin's lifetime. Martin's founding of the College in 1913 put even more strain on the relationship between Martin and the AMA because the AMA claimed that it was the only organization that could unify and represent American medicine and therefore should be the only representative of American physicians.[17]

Even President Woodrow Wilson's appointment of Martin to the Advisory Commission for the Council of National Defense upset the AMA's leadership. They, of course, believed that a representative from the AMA should have received the appointment. Dr. Bevan's attempt to have Martin dismissed from the appointment was unsuccessful, no doubt in part because of Martin's exemplary performance on the commission. In a further attempt to undermine Martin's success, Bevan helped create the journal *Archives of Surgery* as a competitor to *SG&O*. Bevan also attempted to bring the hospital standardization program under AMA control. This endeavor also failed and further provoked Martin.[18]

Although Martin could have been more diplomatic in his approach to contentious issues between the ACS and the AMA, acquiescence to the AMA's requests could and probably would have weakened the ACS as an organization. Placed in the position of being inferior to the AMA, the ACS would never have become the strong advocate for American surgery that it is today. I believe that there are few issues for which Martin fought toe-to-toe with the AMA and won that have not ultimately benefited U.S. and Canadian surgeons. With most of these contentious issues, there was minimal room for compromise if the ACS was going to continue its role as surgery's representative.

Dr. George W. Crile said of Martin's interactions with others whom he considered a challenge to the ACS, "The very characteristics which have made these achievements possible inevitably sometimes seem too aggressive; but in a formative period they are necessary even though they may arouse some antagonism."[19]

In describing Martin's career, Dr. Crile said,

> Franklin Martin has been shy, fearless, imaginative, idealistic, and a dreamer. Long will he be known among the great dreamers in medicine. He dreamed a dream, and the greatest surgical journal in the world was born; he dreamed again and the Clinical Congress

> of Surgeons of North America appeared; he dreamed yet again and the American College of Surgeons came into being.[19]

FEE SPLITTING—A COMPLEX ISSUE

Because of the large discrepancy in fees between physicians in general practice and surgeons, a solution was developed by practicing physicians where the general practitioner received an agreed-upon fee from the surgeon for each patient referral. This highly successful arrangement was called fee splitting, or division of fees, and was prevalent across the country. After an operation, the patient was sent back to the general practitioner, keeping his relationship with the patient and his or her family intact. This arrangement established a mutually beneficial relationship between the two physicians. The downside of this practice was that it reduced competition and potentially could encourage unnecessary surgery.[20]

Many physicians, including many surgeons, thought the practice to be unethical and potentially detrimental to the patient. Fee splitting was one of the first issues addressed at the first formal meeting of the ACS Regents on June 17, 1913. After a long and earnest discussion, Dr. Albert J. Ochsner presented a broad declaration against the division of fees to be signed by all candidates. Dr. Martin then suggested a Fellowship Pledge that was comprehensive in nature.[21] The two were combined into one document, the Fellowship Pledge, that did not use the term "fee splitting" but addressed the issue in detail:

> I pledge myself, so far as I am able, to avoid the sins of selfishness; to shun unwarranted publicity, dishonest money seeking and commercialism as disgraceful to our profession; to refuse utterly all secret money trades with consultants and practitioners; to teach the patient his financial duty to the physician and urge the practitioner to obtain his reward from the patient openly; to make my fees commensurate with the service rendered and with the patient's rights; and to avoid discrediting my associates by taking unwarranted compensation.[22]

Since 1913, the pledge has been revised and changes made in how fee splitting is addressed, but the issue is still addressed in the pledge that Initiates sign today:

> I will take no part in any arrangement or improper financial dealings that induce referral, treatment, or withholding of treatment for reasons other than the patient's welfare.[22]

Among the original goals of the College, the elimination of the division of fees proved one of the most challenging to address. The practice was insidious and difficult to eliminate. Multiple issues needed to be addressed in dealing with the division of fees and any program designed to eliminate the practice had to have a multifaceted approach, which the ACS Regents did not appreciate at the time. The issues were:

- The difficulty of identifying surgeons involved in fee splitting
- The potential liability of the College to be named in defamation suits by the surgeons identified as fee splitters and the difficulties of proving the charge
- The College's lack of any legal authority
- A lack of cooperation from the AMA

Fee splitting was a covert activity that was exceedingly difficult to prove, and in areas where it was widespread, physicians were unwilling to challenge the physicians involved in the activity because of the risk to their livelihood. The College had anticipated that the state and provincial credentials committees would know whether fee splitting was occurring in their area and would deny ACS membership to the implicated surgeons based on the College's Fellowship Pledge and *Bylaws.* Regrettably, the committees were not independent of local politics. Occasionally, politically astute surgeons who practiced fee splitting could still win approval of the local committee. Also, rival surgeons potentially could deprive a qualified surgeon of local committee approval by insinuating that the applicant was involved in fee splitting. The Regents spent immense amounts of time discussing the appeals and counter-appeals of these cases. In the end, fee splitters could lie and still obtain Fellowship, making it difficult for the College to deal with Fellows who continued the practice. The AMA was not opposed to fee splitting and offered no support in dealing with the problem.[23]

By the mid-1920s, the College, using the hospital standardization program, was making some progress in addressing fee splitting. The threat of removing a hospital from the approved list of hospitals or denying approval because of fee splitting was an effective tool. In addition, to decrease the Regents' time spent dealing with appeals, the Board authorized the establishment of state and province judiciary committees. These committees were responsible for informally investigating rumors of unethical or poor conduct and reporting findings to the central office. In addition, the Regents created a Central Judiciary Committee to review the findings of the local committees. Despite these strategies, it would be many years before fee splitting was effectively eliminated.[23]

Dr. Martin was dedicated to the elimination of division of fees, and despite the numerous problems that made its elimination challenging, he continued to seek its extirpation. His dedication is best demonstrated in this quote from him, "The consequences of the division of fees are, first, incompetent medical and surgical service; second, unnecessary surgical operations; and third, the deadening of scientific incentive in the profession."[21]

IMPACT OF BOSTON NEWSPAPER ARTICLE IN 1934 AND MARTIN'S DECLINE

Between meetings at the 1934 Clinical Congress in Boston, Martin gave a brief interview to a *Boston Herald* reporter.[24] The article was published the following day and claimed that Martin had said, "The West is so far ahead of the East as far as surgical progress is concerned that there is simply no comparison"[24] (Figure 14.3). The article alleged that he unfavorably compared Boston surgeons to surgeons in western states, which would have included Illinois and surrounding states at that time. Martin contacted his surgical friends in Boston and denied the remarks attributed to him. Martin wrote a letter to the editor of the newspaper denying that he had made the remarks, but the reporter stood by his story. The College's Executive Committee decided not to release an official reply and instead let the controversy die on its own.

This incident, along with his stroke in 1930 and his recent hospitalization for abdominal pain, raised concerns among close associates about Martin's physical health and his declining mental faculties.

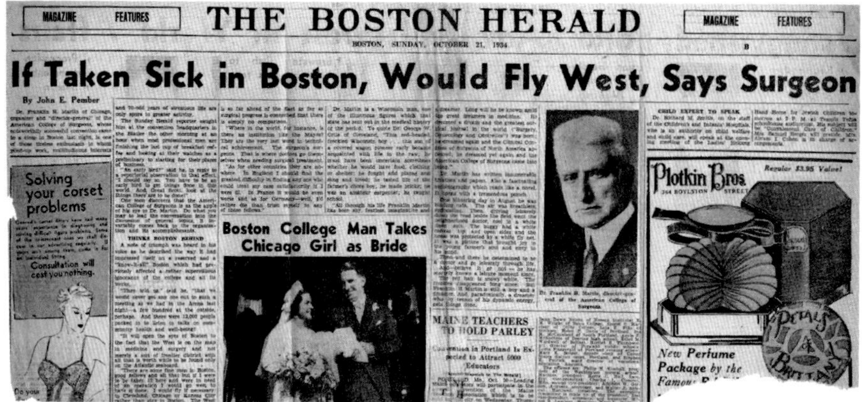
MAGAZINE FEATURES THE BOSTON HERALD MAGAZINE FEATURES

BOSTON, SUNDAY, OCTOBER 21, 1934

If Taken Sick in Boston, Would Fly West, Says Surgeon

By John E. Pember

Boston College Man Takes Chicago Girl as Bride

MAINE TEACHERS TO HOLD PARLEY

14.3. The October 21, 1934, article in The Boston Herald *that created the controversy that led to Martin's decision to consider retiring.*

In view of these concerns, Dr. Crile met with Martin. At the meeting Martin appeared to have agreed to retire, but he later reneged. His friends Drs. William Mayo and Allen Kanavel managed to intercede and convince Martin to begin a transition period at the end of which he would retire. During the transition he would assume the title of Honorary Director-General and be available to mentor his replacement. The day-to-day operations of the College would be managed by a newly appointed Administrative Board. The official date was to be at the conclusion of the Clinical Congress in October 1935, but fate intervened.[25] On February 26, 1935, while at The Biltmore in Phoenix, AZ, Martin suffered an acute myocardial infarction. Initially he was treated in his room at the Biltmore, which was within the standard of care at that time. When he didn't improve, on March 3 he was admitted to St. Joseph's Hospital in Phoenix, where he died on March 7. The Regents decided not to replace Dr. Martin as Director-General of the College, but instead decided to administer the College themselves with an Administrative Board, composed of department managers, Eleanor Grimm, and Marion Farrow, supervising the day-to-day activities of the college. Ms. Farrow, Executive Secretary of the College, was given authority to sign checks and Miss Grimm (as she was always called) was appointed Secretary of the Board of Regents and the Executive Committee of the Board. In reality, Miss Grimm was de facto chief administrative officer of the College for many years.

As excellently outlined by Drs. David Nahrwold and Peter Kernahan in their history of the ACS, the decision to not replace Martin as chief executive officer of the College was not the best path forward. They said,

> ...[the] CEO frequently had to manage conflicts with the government, the AMA, and groups of Fellows in several states who were critical of College policy and leadership. Many Fellows, including some prominent surgical leaders, wanted Martin out;
> ...Not all was well with the Fellows; discontent over College policy existed in all parts of the country. Any other organization of this size and scope that lost its leader would have replaced him.[26]

Martin's replacement would have had a mandate to work with the dissatisfied Fellows, advance the College, and continue to pursue the improvement of surgical care.

Under the designated plan, the Board of Regents would be responsible for the executive's duty of managing the College, in addition to their duty of governance. Authorities in organizational structure could have told them that this plan was not a viable way to go forward. An organization as large and complex as the ACS needed a dedicated, highly organized administrator and leader like Martin to manage its endeavors. Without replacing him with someone with similar abilities, the College was going to struggle in the future. Martin had left the College in good financial shape, with many solid programs. Regrettably, there was no obvious replacement for Martin with similar strengths and abilities. Despite that, the Board of Regents would have served the College more effectively if they had searched for a strong leader with Martin's qualities to steer the College into the future. The Board was divided on how to proceed so they deferred, leaving the College without a Director-General—a decision that would have an impact on the College for years to come.[26]

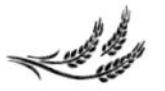

References

1. Martin, F. H. (1933). *The Joy of Living: An Autobiography*, vol. 1 (pp. 441-442). New York, NY: Doubleday, Doran & Co.
2. Nahrwold, D. L., Kernahan, P. J. (2012). *A Century of Surgeons and Surgery: The American College of Surgeons 1913–2012* (pp. 46-47). Chicago, IL: American College of Surgeons.
3. Martin, F. H. (1933). *The Joy of Living: An Autobiography*, vol. 1 (p. 432-434). New York, NY: Doubleday, Doran & Co.
4. Nahrwold, D. L., Kernahan, P. J. (2012). *A Century of Surgeons and Surgery: The American College of Surgeons 1913–2012* (pp. 48-49). Chicago, IL: American College of Surgeons.
5. Ibid., pp. 52-53.
6. Martin, F. H. (1933). *The Joy of Living: An Autobiography*, vol. 1 (p. 449). New York, NY: Doubleday, Doran & Co.
7. Ibid., pp. 450 –452.
8. Crile, G. Foreword. In: Martin, F. H. (1933). *The Joy of Living: An Autobiography*, vol. 1 (pp. xiii –xiv), New York, NY: Doubleday, Doran & Co.
9. Martin, F. H. (1933). *The Joy of Living: An Autobiography*, vol. 1 (pp. 453-455). New York, NY: Doubleday, Doran & Co.
10. Nahrwold, D. L., Kernahan, P. J. (2012). *A Century of Surgeons and Surgery: The American College of Surgeons 1913–2012* (pp. 57-59). Chicago, IL: American College of Surgeons.
11. Nahrwold, D. L., Kernahan, P. J. (2012). *A Century of Surgeons and Surgery: The American College of Surgeons 1913–2012* (pp. 69-71). Chicago, IL: American College of Surgeons.
12. Ibid., pp. 71-73.
13. Ibid., p. 67-68.
14. Ibid., p. 68
15. Ibid., pp. 34-36.
16. Ibid., pp. 75-80.
17. Ibid., p. 77.
18. Ibid., p. 35.
19. Crile, G. (1935). Franklin H. Martin and the American College of Surgeons. *Bull Am Coll Surg*, (20), 52.
20. Nahrwold, D. L., Kernahan, P. J. (2012). *A Century of Surgeons and Surgery: The American College of Surgeons 1913–2012* (p. 7). Chicago, IL: American College of Surgeons.

21. Martin, F. H. (1933). *The Joy of Living: An Autobiography*, vol. 1 (p. 432-434). New York, NY: Doubleday, Doran & Co.
22. American College of Surgeons Archives. The Evolution of the Fellowship Pledge. Available at: www.facs.org/about-acs/archives/pasthighlights/pledge. Accessed August 10, 2020.
23. Nahrwold, D. L., Kernahan, P. J. (2012). *A Century of Surgeons and Surgery: The American College of Surgeons 1913–2012* (pp. 50-51). Chicago, IL: American College of Surgeons.
24. Pember, J. F. (1934, October 21). If taken sick in Boston, would fly west, says surgeon. *The Boston Herald*, sec. B, p. 1.
25. Nahrwold, D. L., Kernahan, P. J. (2012). *A Century of Surgeons and Surgery: The American College of Surgeons 1913–2012* (pp. 89-91). Chicago, IL: American College of Surgeons.
26. Ibid., pp. 91-98.

Chapter 15

Trips Back to Wisconsin

-on moved on ~~was~~
that the Corliss house ~~was~~ brought
Invitations on Sunday had Every bo-
claim on the big bend.
the raising on Saturday. Volunteer
~~hands~~ were busy from all the neig- [adjoin-]
the week, felling trees, and hewing ~~the~~
-ts shape for the new house. Early
-g of Saturday a dozen or more sli-
and boys were on hand to construc-
house. A cellar had been dug in th-
~~fields~~ ready to be encased with ston-
-elm logs had been sunk in ben-
reached a bed of solid clay beneath th-
-il, lumber had been brought fro-
-ow mill and a fine lot of dry
been contributed by generous neighbor-
-ers ~~oxen~~ ready to compete with S-
sturdy oxen that had been brou-
neighbors.

Jean Martin by common cons-
-man for the day. No time was [of the gang]
all directions came the great logs
iron chains about their necks a-
... of the faithful oxen

Summer of 1899

Before 1918, Martin appears to have returned to Wisconsin only occasionally to visit family and conduct family business. Just one of these trips, in the summer of 1899, was well documented, and is recounted in a series of photographs located in the ACS Archives (Figure 15.1). During this trip he visited members of the Martin family in Oconomowoc, the Carlin family in Watertown, and friends at the site of the family homesteads on the Rock River.

August 1918

On August 22, 1918, on his way to the annual Tri-State (Wisconsin, Illinois, and Iowa) Medical Society meeting in Madison, WI, Martin visited his sister Nettie (Mrs. Jeanette Martin Rust Humburch) and his Uncle Addison Carlin (Uncle Ad) in Watertown (Figure 15.2), after which he and Uncle Ad went to Oconomowoc to visit Martin's Aunt Millie (Mrs. Luther Hatch, his father's sister), whom he not seen in 20 years. He remembered Aunt Millie as a great talker and entertainer, as was her husband. He recollected playing baseball, going to the local swimming hole with his cousins Alfred and Charles Hatch, and the wonderful food that Aunt Millie served the family.[1] To his surprise, many other relatives from his father's family were in attendance.

Starting in the 1870s, the Oconomowoc area, with its magnificent lakes and picturesque surroundings, had become a destination for wealthy families from all corners of the U.S., especially nearby Chicago, where the summer heat could be unpleasant. In the following years many of these families, including the Montgomery Wards of Chicago, built homes on the shores of Lac La Belle and other area lakes until the waters were surrounded by large mansions with magnificent grounds and gardens.

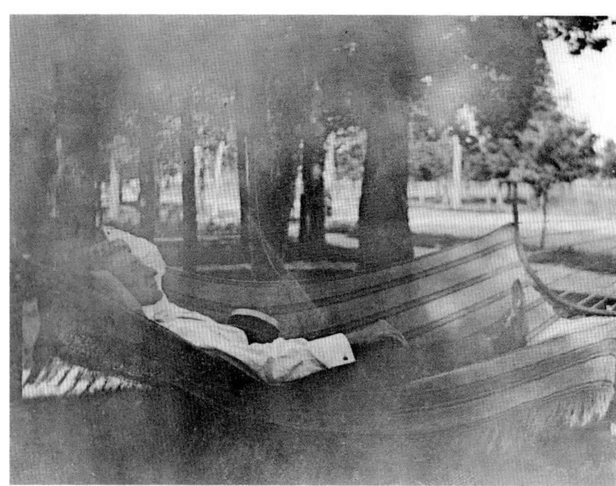

Figure 15.1. The Martins' 1899 trip to Wisconsin.

15.1a. Martin relaxing in hammock during visit to Oconomowoc.

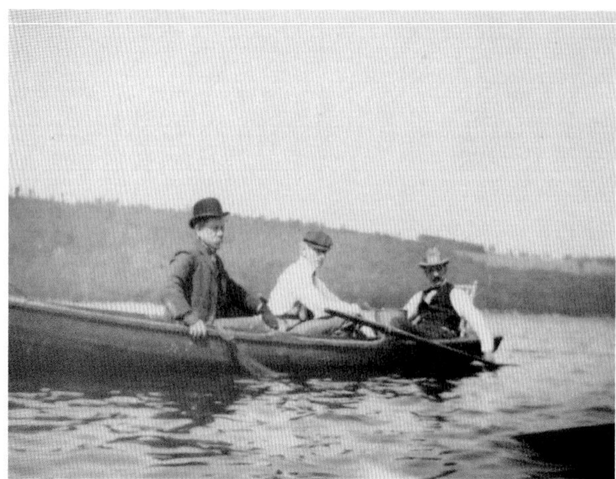

15.1b. Martin (center) and friends boating on the Rock River in Ixonia.

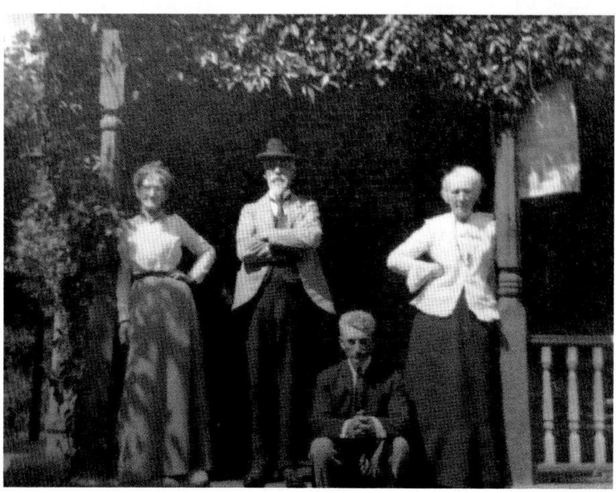

15.1c. From left: Aunt Mary Carlin, Uncle Addison Carlin, Franklin, and an unidentified friend or family member on the porch of Uncle Ad's home in Watertown.

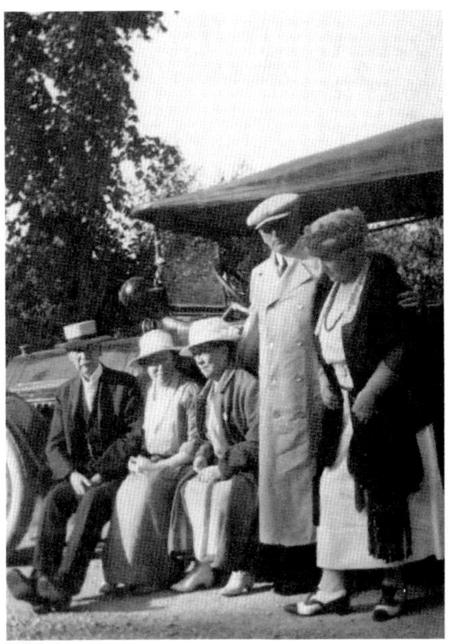

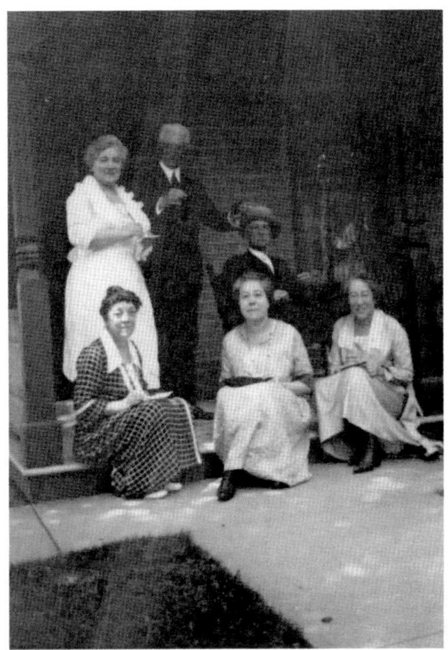

15.2. Franklin and Isabelle's 1918 trip to Wisconsin.

15.2a. (left). From left: Martin's Uncle Addison Carlin, Katherine Harris, Isabelle Martin, Franklin Martin, and Jeanette Humburch (Martin's sister).

15.2b. (right). Front row: Isabelle Martin, Katherine Harris, and Caroline Harris. Back row: Jeanette Humburch, Martin, and Uncle Addison Carlin.

Martin wrote warmly about the opportunity to drive around the wonderful lakes and countryside of Oconomowoc. The drive brought back wonderful memories of his early life in these glorious surroundings. He said of returning, "It seems like a dream of a pure paradise."[2] All the landmarks of his youth were gone, he said, "But the hill, the river and the same blessed memories were there and we could point out in imagination and memory where the dear things once were."[2]

On returning to Watertown, Martin, Isabelle, Nettie, and their friend Katherine Harris proceeded to Madison to attend the annual banquet of the Tri-State Medical Society, where Martin would be giving an address. At this time, Martin was still a member of the Advisory Commission of the Council of National Defense, so he spoke about the Volunteer Medical Service Corps and urged the physicians in the audience to enroll in the Corps. After the meeting, they drove back to Watertown, where they stayed overnight before returning to Chicago.[3]

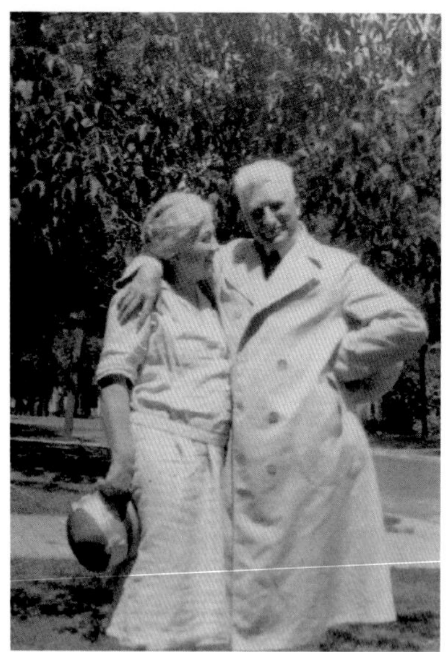
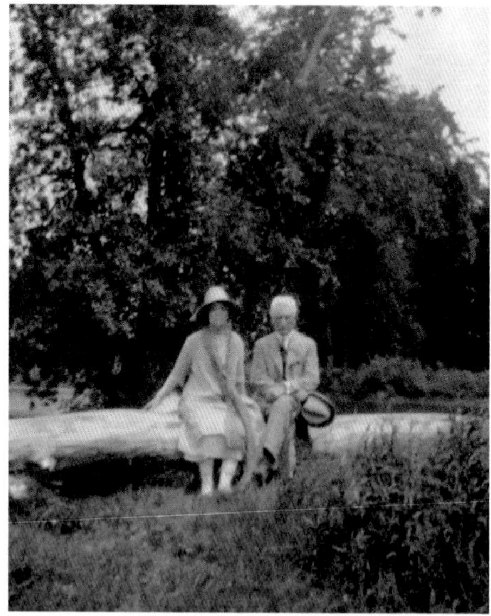

15.3. Franklin's and Isabelle's trips back to Wisconsin in the 1920s and 1930s.
15.3a (left). Martin and his sister Jeanette (Nettie) Martin Humburch.
15.3b (right). Martin and Isabelle on the Rock River.

1920s and 1930s

Between 1925 and his death in 1935, Martin and Isabelle returned to Wisconsin on several occasions to visit family and friends and enjoy the surroundings where he'd lived out his early life. During these trips they visited Ixonia, Watertown, Oconomowoc, and other areas of significance to him. He seemed to want to show his wife and friends why remembering his times in Wisconsin brought him such joy (Figure 15.3). Three times in his autobiography Martin uses the phrase "joy of living," which is the title of the book, and in all three instances it was in reference to his life in Wisconsin. The first mention related to the impact on his life of his upbringing in Wisconsin,

> The train wended its way through the lake region where we had been born, had learned to play, to work, and to swim, and had developed strong bodies and clear minds.... Our young souls were filled with joy; and this joy of living was enhanced by anticipation of the immediate future....[4]

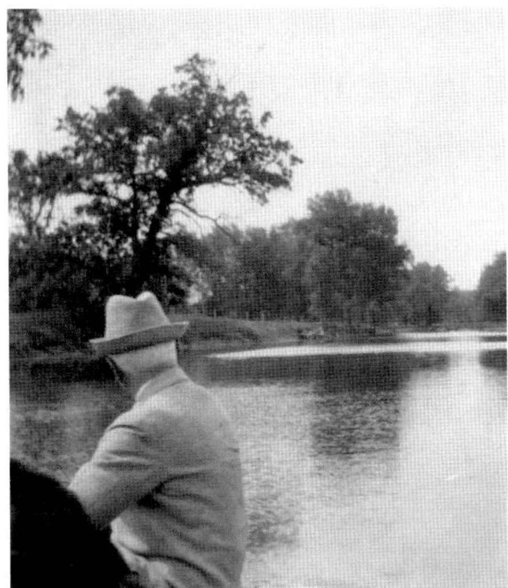
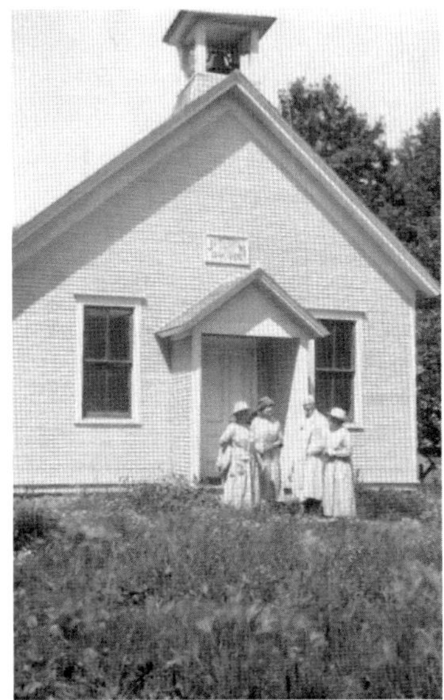

15.4. Places of special importance to Martin that he visited in the 1920s and 1930s.

15.4a (left). Martin boating on the Rock River.

15.4b (right). Martin, Isabelle, and their friends Katherine and Caroline Harris in front of the Oak Grove School, where Martin taught.

The second was about his work in the brickyard,

> Young 'Dock' had come back to work with his cousins and to enjoy life in an environment of honest, God-fearing people who were full of the joy of living. Work was a necessity, and in the eyes of these honest folk no man was meaner than he who shirked his daily task. It was an outdoor life, and the men with whom I worked did not tire and were ever ready for a wholesome frolic. Their recreation was fishing, hunting, baseball, picnics, visiting, and buggy-riding with their best girls.[5]

The third was in reference to his attending Cubs' baseball games with Isabelle:

> ...an intangible something brought health, extreme joy of living, and 'pep' that I had not enjoyed since my labors in the brickyard and on the farm.[6]

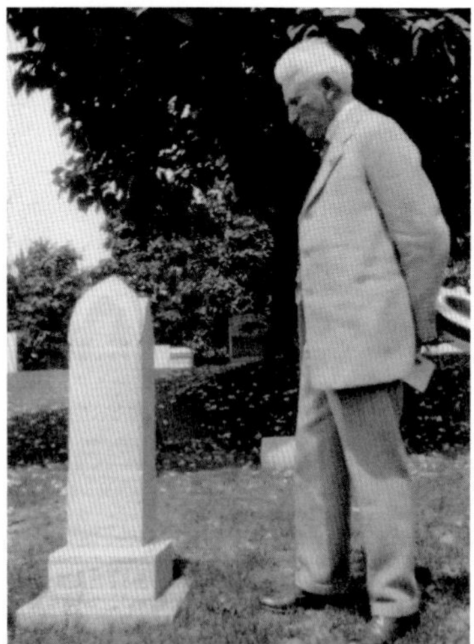

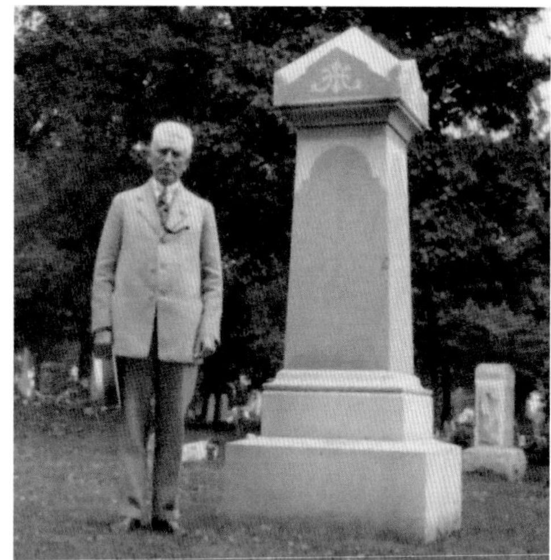

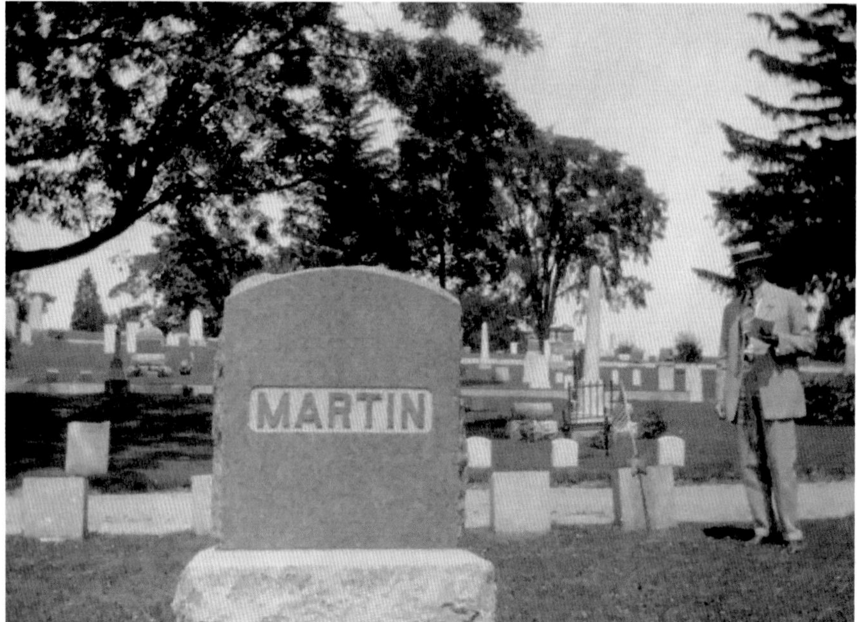

15.5. Martin visiting the Martin and Carlin family monuments monuments in the 1930s.

15.5a (top left). Martin viewing the monument of his grandparents William and Caroline (Phelps) Martin in La Belle Cemetery, Oconomowoc, WI.

15.5b (top right). Martin next to the Carlin family monument in Oak Hill Cemetery, Watertown, WI.

15.5c (bottom). Martin next to his parents' monuments, La Belle Cemetery.

When describing his time spent in the fields at his Grandfather Carlin's farm, Martin said, "I soon found that it was not irksome, and now count among the happiest of my life the days and weeks spent in the fields, the woods, and the pasture, with a drove of cattle and my ever-faithful companion, Major"—his grandfather's intelligent shepherd dog.[7]

Putting all these quotes in perspective, one can see that, although Martin had an unbelievably successful career, when he looked back on his life it was his early years in Wisconsin that brought the most joy to him later in life.

Martin's routine as a physician, surgeon, and administrator did not allow him the opportunity to be active during the workday, so he developed a routine of taking long walks almost daily, and he began playing golf in 1898 at the age of 41. These pastimes gave him the opportunity to exercise and be outdoors, which was important to him and necessary for both his physical and psychological well-being. He described using the time he spent on these long walks to think through issues he was facing at work and bring some clarity to their possible resolution. One friend described being asked to join Martin on a walk in the hopes that they could resolve an issue of mutual concern.[8]

Martin said of golf: "Many of the leaders in our civilization first saw the light of day in a country or farmland home; and as a counterbalance to their strenuous labors and their confinement, golf took them back to the freedom of Nature."[9] The joy of living to Martin was not in his surgical career and his numerous accomplishments as an administrator, but rather in his upbringing and work in the outdoors. That is not to say that his accomplishments as a physician were not tremendously rewarding to him; they just did not bring the same joy to his life as his work with his family members in the brickyard and in the fields during the harvesting of grain. So, it is no surprise that late in life he wanted to return to Wisconsin to relive those experiences and share his feelings with his wife and friends.

The itineraries for the trips to Wisconsin varied. They visited family, the family homesteads where he had grown up, the Rock River where he had played as a youth, the Oak Grove School where he had taught, the Fulmer brickyard where he had labored, and many other sites (Figure 15.4). He also visited the family monuments at the cemeteries where his parents, grandparents, and other family members were buried (Figure 15.5). In July 1935, a few months after Martin died, Isabelle returned to Wisconsin to visit his family.

Despite a phenomenally successful career that gave him tremendous satisfaction, late in life Martin seemed to derive a deep-seated pleasure from reminiscing about his days in the brickyard and fields and his upbringing in the great Wisconsin outdoors. One can assume that returning to Wisconsin brought into perspective the importance of his life experiences during his first 20 years and their significant impact on his subsequent success.

REFERENCES

1. Martin, F. H. Unpublished diary. 1918, August 22. In: *Franklin H. Martin Collection,* Archives of the American College of Surgeons, Chicago, IL.
2. Martin, F. H. Unpublished diary. 1918, August 23. In: *Franklin H. Martin Collection,* Archives of the American College of Surgeons, Chicago, IL.
3. Martin, F. H. (1933). *The Joy of Living: An Autobiography,* vol. 2 (pp. 360-361). New York, NY: Doubleday, Doran & Co.
4. Martin, F. H. (1933). *The Joy of Living: An Autobiography,* vol. 1 (p. 128). New York, NY: Doubleday, Doran & Co.
5. Ibid., p. 149
6. Ibid., p. 318.
7. Ibid., pp. 43-44.
8. Miller, C. J. (1935). Franklin H. Martin—the friend. *Bull Am Coll Surg,* 20(2), 45.
9. Martin, F. H. (1933). *The Joy of Living: An Autobiography,* vol. 1 (pp. 371-373). New York, NY: Doubleday, Doran & Co.

Chapter 16

The Lifelong Process of Becoming a Leader

oon noised a[bout] ~~[struck]~~ thought t[hat]
that the Corliss house had b[rought]
Missions on Sunday had. Every bo[dy]
claim on the big bend. Volunteer[s]
the raising on Saturday. Volunteer[s]
~~hands~~ were busy from all the neig[hbors]
the week, felling trees, hewing and adjoin[ing] ~~the~~
ir shape for the new house. Early
g of Saturday a dozen or more st[rong men]
and boys were on hand to construc[t]
house, ~~A~~ cellar had been dug in t[he]
~~[struck]~~ ready to be encased with ston[e]
ian logs had been sunk in ben[eath]
eached a bed of solid clay beneath the
il, lumber had been brought from
w mill and a fine lot of dry
been contributed by generous neighbors
ven ~~[struck]~~ ready to complete with se[veral]
sturdy oxen that had been brou[ght]
neighbors.
Tom Indian by common cons[ent]
oseman of the gang for the day. No time was
all directions came the great logs
iron chains about their necks a[nd]
by of the faithful oxen [and] cheery

As described in previous chapters, Franklin Martin's early life in rural Wisconsin had a significant impact on the development of his leadership and organizational abilities. These strengths made it feasible for him to develop into a great leader. When he was young, he often sought employment to help with family expenses and to pay for his own needs, and these pursuits also helped to build his character (Figure 16.1).

His background contributed to his strength of character, self-confidence, and ability to follow his vision when others might have hesitated. When Martin was convinced that his approach to an issue was correct, he was resolute in advocating for his solution. Unlike many administrators and leaders, often he would move forward without waiting for support from others, and almost never appointed a committee to evaluate an idea or project; he developed his own strategy and only sought assistance when he was ready to put his plan into action. When Martin envisioned and initiated a project like the founding of the American College of Surgeons, he often proceeded with the encouragement of only a few of his contemporaries. An astute organizer, even under difficult circumstances he didn't procrastinate. Perhaps most importantly, he had the discipline and stamina to maintain his focus and forge ahead, undistracted by issues he deemed inconsequential.

Martin was the type of leader who inspired confidence in those who worked with him, earning their steadfast dedication and loyalty. His major achievements make up an impressive list (Figure 16.2).

His close friend Dr. J. Bentley Squier described Martin as "a man who as he matured became the greatest organizer which the past fifty years of medicine has produced."[1] He went on to say,

> There are many qualities common to those among men who leave their names conspicuously high on the rolls of achievement of the era in which they lived. Oft included in these are the circumstance of lowly birth and early struggles against privations combined with integrity of mind, indomitable will, and other steadfast qualities.[1]

I couldn't agree more with this statement. Even his friends understood where his strong character originated.

Early Life Experiences Start Martin on the Path to Later Achievements

Franklin's father died in the Civil War in 1862 when Martin was five years old. Losing a parent at such a young age certainly had a profound impact on him. In the ensuing years, he felt it was his responsibility to contribute money for family necessities. For example, when bargaining with his Grandfather Carlin over his compensation for work on the Carlin farm, he requested cash, in his words, "to contribute it toward things that had heretofore been provided."[2] Thus, at an early age he demonstrated a burgeoning self-reliance and a strong need to behave responsibly.[2]

Beginning at age five, Martin had daily chores to do at home, as well as when visiting Grandfather Carlin's farm, his Uncle George and Uncle William Fulmer's farms, and his Uncle Adolphus Guilder's home. He was expected to perform his chores in a timely and proper fashion, which imbued him with a sense of responsibility at a young age.[3,4]

At age nine, Martin began working summers on the Carlin and Fulmer farms in earnest. Working in the fields and caring for the livestock, eventually without direct supervision, he gained self-confidence and a sense of discipline, performing complicated tasks correctly and efficiently. He realized then that learning simple techniques ultimately would make complex tasks easier to perform.[5,6]

Growing Sense of Enterprise and Industry

After spending his ninth summer in 1866 working on the Carlin farm, Martin requested, in addition to money, an ewe that was expected to produce two lambs. Martin parlayed the one sheep into nine and sold them at a nice profit.[7] Martin said of this experience: "I had learned to assume responsibilities, to transact small financial deals, and had industriously busied myself…."[8]

Over the next few years Franklin had many jobs. At age 12, he expanded his weeding of the family garden into a small but successful neighborhood weeding business. In this case, his organized, diligent,

FIGURE 16.1

FRANKLIN MARTIN'S WORK HISTORY BEFORE BECOMING A PHYSICIAN

AGE	EMPLOYMENT
9	Hired hand on Grandfather Carlin's farm, Watertown, WI
12–13	Hired hand on Carlin and Fulmer farms, Oconomowoc, WI
13–14	Gardener and school janitor in Oconomowoc, WI
14–15	Handyman and supervisor in Uncle Adolphus Gilder's milling plant, Minneapolis, MN
16	Janitor at Elroy Seminary, Elroy, WI
16	Schoolteacher at Mauston Public School, Mauston, WI
17	Laborer in Fulmer brickyard, Oconomowoc, WI
18	Schoolteacher at Bushman School, Ixonia, WI
19	Farm laborer at Russell farm, Concord, WI
19	Laborer in Fulmer brickyard
19–20	Farm laborer on Carlin farm
20	Farm laborer on Fulmer farm
21	Schoolteacher, Oak Grove School, Oak Grove, WI
22	Caregiver for Mr. William Hickling, Chicago, IL

and thorough approach to weeding gained him a sound reputation and lucrative work.[9] When he was 13 to 14 years old, the family fell on hard times. As would be expected from someone with his character, Franklin contributed by becoming the substitute, and eventually the head, janitor at the village school. His duties required Franklin to be meticulous and methodical. It must have improved his self-confidence when he succeeded in fine fashion.[10] He had a similar experience at the age of 17 as the school janitor at the Elroy Seminary.[11] Soon thereafter, Franklin began a business with a school friend, cutting and splitting firewood for neighbors. To compete for this work, the boys had to complete a strenu-

Figure 16.2

Highlights of Franklin Martin's Career

1882–1916	Clinical practice of obstetrics and gynecology, Chicago, IL
1883	Co-organized the Chicago South-Side Medico-Social Society
1889	Co-founded the Post-Graduate Medical School and Hospital of Chicago
1905	Founded the journal *Surgery, Gynecology & Obstetrics* (name later changed to *Journal of the American College of Surgeons*)
1910	Founded the Clinical Congress of the Surgeons of North America (now the Clinical Congress of the American College of Surgeons)
1913	Founded the American College of Surgeons (ACS)
1913	Created the hospital standardization program
1913–1917	General Secretary of the ACS
1916	Appointed by President Woodrow Wilson to the Advisory Commission of the Council of National Defense in preparation for World War I
1917–1922	Secretary-General of the ACS
1922–1935	Director-General of the ACS
1920	Created state and provincial chapters of the ACS and established sectional meetings
1920, 1923	Traveled to Central and South America as a representative of the ACS to help establish a relationship with surgeons in those areas
1928–1929	Twelfth President of the ACS

ous task with efficiency and precision.[12] Although the money he earned was his to spend as he wished, Martin always requested his mother's advice when deciding how to best use his sparse earnings. Usually, she recommended the purchase of something practical—imbuing her son with a healthy pragmatism.[13]

Taking on More Responsibility with Imagination and Energy

At age 15, Franklin worked as an apprentice millwright at his Uncle Adolphus Guilder's flour milling and manufacturing plant in Minneapolis. While acting as a handyman, he mastered the principles and mechanics of the machinery, and helped installed new flour purifiers in local mills. He was given increased responsibility, occasionally in a supervisory position, and he took on new duties when the factory expanded. In the grueling environment, he learned to be precise, thorough, and increasingly self-confident.[14] As described in Chapter 3, Franklin obtained white hickory blocks from his family in Wisconsin to make high-quality pick handles for the mill's stone pickers who redressed the stones used to grind the wheat. Franklin perceived a need, designed a way to fulfill it and, in the process, make a significant amount of money. His background of performing manual labor with his father and his uncles contributed to his insight and ability to solve this practical problem.[15]

Expanding His World by Teaching and Hard Work

At age 17, Franklin taught at a small school near Mauston, WI. There he used the carpentry and masonry skills learned from his stepfather to perform repairs to the school. He took inspiration from the few students he felt he had encouraged. Martin used his organizational and practical skills to guide his teaching, and even to fight the brushfires that occasionally crept near the school.[16]

At age 18, and again at ages 19 and 21, Martin worked in his Uncle George Fulmer's brickyard—a job that turned out to be as strenuous as any he ever performed. Adapting quickly, he continued to develop as a disciplined, hardworking, and organized laborer. He learned the importance of adhering to a high standard and to be a valuable team member in an egalitarian work environment, which strengthened his self-confidence and character.[17-19]

At age 19, Martin taught at the Bushman School. Martin outlined and strictly enforced the rules; as a result, the formerly disruptive children learned discipline. He instituted elocution and memorization exercises to divert the energy of the robust children. Although Martin's major frustration with his teaching career was his belief that he had not imparted significant amounts of new knowledge to his students, his vision and thoughtfulness resulted in a scholarly atmosphere at the school, and the community applauded his accomplishments.[20]

At the end of the school term, Martin worked on the Russell Farm in Concord. The work was strenuous, but he adapted rapidly and said of his experience working for Mr. Arthur Russell,

> What was more wholesome than a useful occupation in the open air, with pleasant surroundings, and with a mind filled for the first time with the wonders of wonders that the sages of the world, too, had considered worthy of their greatest efforts in philosophy, in eloquence, in poem and in song?[21]

At age 22, after his second year of medical school, Martin taught at the Oak Grove School, and again he prospered. The older students in the class, who were only slightly younger than Franklin, requested that he teach them new, more advanced subjects, and although Franklin was unfamiliar with some of the topics, he developed inventive teaching techniques, to both his own and the students' satisfaction.[22]

Envisioning a Professional Future

As discussed in Chapter 4, although Franklin loved doing useful work outdoors in pleasant surroundings, he did not relish the thought of performing heavy labor for the rest of his life. It was then that he decided to become a doctor. He envisioned a professional future for himself and proceeded to make it happen. When he finally completed his training and went into the practice of medicine, Martin continued his habit of hard work and approached his duties with vigor. To compensate for the lack of strenuous, open-air activity, he took long walks almost daily for the remainder of his life.

Even as a 19-year-old student of Dr. Spalding in 1876, lodging with his grandparents, Martin helped with the household and farm chores every morning before going to the doctor's office. By this time, Martin's strong character and willingness to work hard, along with the ease with which he accepted responsibility, meant that he could ably organize and carry out his daily chores—as he had done since he was five years old.[23]

Under Dr. Spalding's tutelage, Martin demonstrated an uncanny ability to learn anatomy and recite it perfectly. He approached learning the subject with the same tenacity that he approached teaching, farming, brickmaking, and all his many jobs. After completing his studies with Dr. Spalding, Franklin again worked at his Uncle William Fulmer's farm. Besides the routine chores, he was placed in charge of a large hop field, something he had never done before. By this time in his life, Martin had enough discipline and responsibility to plan, organize, and complete any task and to achieve an excellent outcome—so he efficiently cultivated and harvested the crop.[24]

Martin's final job before beginning his medical career was caring for Mr. William Hickling, a wealthy but basically bedridden man. His pay was to be $5 a day, more than twice the rate Martin had ever earned. He learned again the importance of reputation, because a medical school professor had recommended him for the job. One of the tremendous benefits of this position was Martin's exposure to Mr. Hickling's extensive library, which he appreciated for the remainder of his life.[25]

MARTIN'S COLLEAGUES PAY TRIBUTE TO HIS QUALITIES

Martin's friends and colleagues extolled his personal qualities in the obituaries published in the *Bulletin of the American College of Surgeons* in 1935, and it's interesting to compare the characteristics that they ascribed to him with the ones described in previous chapters—qualities he began to develop in his younger years. Dr. William R. Cubbins called him sturdy and industrious.[26] Dr. Frederic A. Besley said he had clarity of thought, directness of expression, and made logical deductions and sound conclusions. He described him as a dynamic force with untiring spirit and said that no barrier he faced was unsurmountable. He believed he had great vision, courage, and a will to succeed. Lastly, he believed that as an organizer Martin had untiring energy and industry.[27]

Dr. C. Jeff Miller praised Martin as a leader of men and a versatile organizer. He also described him as having courage, fearlessness, resourcefulness, and sound judgment, and called him a constructive and creative dreamer.[28] Dr. Allen B. Kanavel called Martin an idealist and said he arrived at logical conclusions much more rapidly than his peers, who would eventually come around to his point of view.[29]

Dr. George W. Crile perceived Martin as having a lively imagination, wisdom, and courage. He had the ability to inspire unfailing loyalty when he needed support for a cause. He believed Martin had rare executive ability and that no other man could have equaled his performance in establishing and shaping the ACS. Crile believed—as I do—that although in some circumstances Martin appeared too aggressive and unyielding, in formative times such a stance was necessary. In Crile's words, "The very characteristics which have made these achievements possible inevitably sometimes seemed too aggressive; but in a formative period they are necessary even though they may arouse some antagonism."[30] If not for his unwavering support of ACS policies, even under tremendous pressure to relent, the ACS would not be the robust organization that it is to this day. Crile also called Martin fearless and idealistic, saying that he was one of the greatest visionaries in medicine of his time.[30]

Looking back over these times in Martin's life, Dr. Bentley J. Squier said of him, "We see him in his youth with the spirit of D'Artagnan, recognizing no obstacles as insurmountable and ready for life's adventures with a happy heart." He added,

> Martin had the unusual combination of not alone being an organizer, but having the added quality of being able to make his organizations functionate peculiarly well after he had built them.... Martin had an extraordinary ability to appreciate immediately which were the most important details of any problem and to recognize instantly the right thing to do under adverse conditions.[1]

Admiral Cary T. Grayson wrote of Martin that he was an administrative genius with vision. He said that without Martin the U.S. military during World War I would have lacked the necessary medical resources. As he had done with the ACS, after envisioning and setting a wartime course for the Medical Corps, Martin was tireless in seeing his projects through to a successful conclusion.[31]

Dr. J. Bentley Squier also declared that Martin was the greatest organizer in medicine of his era, saying,

> There are, however, deeper influences which must predetermine a man's ultimate worth, and nature having endowed Franklin Martin with the rugged qualities of strong character gave him also a fineness of sensibility which tempered his thoughts with keen discernment and his judgment with unfailing fairness and justice.[1]

He said of Martin that his skills and personality gave him the ability to create an organization that truly worked. Martin had the perception to appreciate the important details of an issue and could recognize the right way to proceed, even under adverse circumstances.[1]

Dr. William Mayo said of him, "Dr. Martin possesses certain impressive qualities, perhaps the most conspicuously courage, which with knowledge and character laid the foundation for the respect and admiration held for him by his confrères."[32]

Dr. John M. T. Finney, a Johns Hopkins University surgeon and the first President of the American College of Surgeons, said of Martin,

> He was in many respects a remarkable man, a born organizer, a man of vision and a good deal of an individualist, as men of this type always are, but with it all a man with whom one could not be closely associated for any length of time without coming to respect and admire his many excellent qualities.[33]

To reiterate Dr. George W. Crile's remarks about Martin:

> All through his life, and despite every disguise, Franklin Martin has been shy, fearless, imaginative, idealistic and a dreamer. Long will he be known among the great dreamers in medicine. He dreamed a dream, and the greatest surgical journal in the world was born; he dreamed again and the Clinical Congress of the Surgeons of North America appeared; he dreamed yet again and the American College of Surgeons came into being.[34]

When one looks at the characteristics that Martin developed in his formative years, and the characteristics his peers and friends ascribed to him throughout his career as a physician, there is obviously a strong match—which is why I believe that so much of what Martin achieved was because of his rural upbringing.

References

1. Squier, J. B. (1935). Franklin H. Martin—the man. *Bull Am Coll Surg*, 20(2), 56-57.
2. Martin, F. H. (1933). *The Joy of Living: An Autobiography*, vol. 1 (p. 46). New York, NY: Doubleday, Doran & Co.
3. Ibid., p. 31.
4. Ibid., p. 55.
5. Ibid., pp. 39-45.
6. Ibid., p. 58.
7. Ibid., pp. 45-47.
8. Ibid., pp. 53-54.
9. Ibid., pp. 59-60.
10. Ibid., p. 61.
11. Ibid., p. 78.
12. Ibid., pp. 61-62.
13. Ibid., pp. 62-63.
14. Ibid., pp. 70-76.
15. Ibid., pp. 71-72.
16. Ibid., pp. 82-86.
17. Ibid., pp. 91-100.
18. Ibid., pp. 117-118.
19. Ibid., pp. 149-150.
20. Ibid., pp. 108-111.
21. Ibid., pp. 112-114.
22. Ibid., pp. 165-170.
23. Ibid., pp. 118-119.
24. Ibid., pp. 124-125.
25. Ibid., pp. 187-195.
26. Cubbins, W. R. (1935). Franklin H. Martin. *Bull Am Coll Surg*, 20(2), 39-40.

27. Besley, F. A. (1935). Franklin H. Martin—the surgeon. *Bull Am Coll Surg*, 20(2), 41-43.
28. Miller, C. J. (1935). Franklin H. Martin—the friend. *Bull Am Coll Surg*, 20(2), 44-46.
29. Kanavel, A. B. (1935). Franklin H. Martin and *Surgery, Gynecology and Obstetrics*. *Bull Am Coll Surg*, 20(2), 47-49.
30. Crile, G. (1935). Franklin H. Martin and The American College of Surgeons. *Bull Am Coll Surg*, 120(2), 50-52.
31. Grayson, C. T. (1935). Franklin H. Martin and The Great War. *Bull Am Coll Surg*, 20(2), 53-55.
32. Mayo, W. J. Foreword. In Martin, F. H. (1933). *The Joy of Living: An Autobiography*, vol. 1 (p. xi). New York, NY: Doubleday, Doran & Co.
33. Finney, J. M. T. (1940). *A Surgeons Life: The Autobiography of J. M. T. Finney* (p. 133). New York, NY: G. P. Putnam's Sons.
34. Crile, G. W. Foreword. In Martin, F. H. (1933). *The Joy of Living: An Autobiography*, vol. 1 (p. xiii). New York, NY: Doubleday, Doran & Co.

Chapter 17

Other Successful Surgeons Who Benefited from a Rural Upbringing

oon noised ... that the Corbins house ... bought ... Irishes on Sunday had ... Every ... claim on the big bend. ... the raising on Saturday. Volunteers ... were busy from all the neig... the week, felling trees, hewing and adjustin... the shape for the new house. Early ... of Saturday a dozen or more ... and boys were on hand to construct ... house. A cellar had been dug in ... ready to be encased with stone ... logs had been sunk in ... reached a bed of solid clay beneath the ... lumber had been brought from ... mill and a fine lot of ... been contributed by generous neighbors ... ready to compete with ... sturdy oxen that had been brou... neighbors.

Irish boy common ... of the year for the day, no time ... all devotions came the great log ... chains about their necks ... of the faithful oxen ...

Franklin Martin was not the only surgeon of his era who benefited from a rural upbringing. To this day, surgeons raised on family farms speak warmly of the positive impact of farm life and a rural background on their professional careers. The surgeons and their biographers often describe their character in the same terms I've used to describe Martin. Although working on a modern, mechanized farm is less grueling than farming in the late 1800s and early 1900s, farming still is a labor-intensive and rigorous occupation that can require the entire family to work long hours, especially during the planting and harvesting seasons.

The benefits of growing up in a rural environment can be broad and impactful. I recall speaking with a surgery resident who, after spending all night in the intensive care unit caring for a very ill patient, explained to me that this was not the first time he had been up all night with a sick patient—but those earlier patients had four legs, not two. He compared answering to the attending surgeon in the morning with answering to his farmer father and pointed out that the two experiences weren't vastly different.

Following are examples of other prominent surgeons who profited from their rural upbringing.

Dr. John B. Murphy

John Benjamin (J. B.) Murphy (Figure 17.1) was born December 21, 1857, in Appleton, WI, into a hard-working farm family. John, his two brothers, and his father farmed 128 acres of fertile land. They toiled from sunup to sundown—plowing, sowing, harvesting, and, when time allowed, clearing trees. John and his brothers also trapped muskrats, rabbits, squirrels, and bobcats. They hunted wolves for the $5 to $10 bounty for the hides.

Murphy's parents made sure that all the children received a solid education. Murphy quoted his mother as saying, "If you are educated, there are no man's achievements which you cannot equal or excel, provided you have industry and integrity and are temperate."[1] Murphy learned from his father Michael that indolence was the most frequent cause of failure in a man. Murphy's biographer, Loyal Davis, said of his parent's influence on John and his brothers,

> Whereas Michael [Murphy's father] taught their children the virtue and the necessity of courage, industry, determination of purpose, and above all else discipline in the husbandry of small resources—the value of which cannot be denied—Ann emphasized the intellectual limitations of herself and their father.[1]

After high school, Murphy passed the teacher's examination and, like Franklin Martin, taught at a local school before losing interest and deciding to become a doctor. After precepting with a local physician, he attended Rush Medical College, Chicago, and interned at Cook County Hospital. He trained further in Europe and returned to Chicago to practice medicine and surgery. Within a few years he became recognized as a leader in American surgery and eventually gained international prominence. William Mayo called him a surgical genius. Murphy became a leader in abdominal surgery and a founding member of the American College of Surgeons (ACS). Like Martin, Murphy's rural upbringing helped him develop into a hard-working, highly dedicated surgeon.[1]

Dr. Nicholas Senn

In 1852, when he was eight years old, Nicholas Senn's family moved from Switzerland to the rural community of Ashford, WI (Figure 17.2). Like Martin and Murphy, after graduating from high school he taught school for two terms. He enjoyed nature and loved to study the flora of his surroundings. He graduated from the Chicago Medical College in 1868, interned at Cook County Hospital, and returned to Elmore, WI, to practice medicine. In 1877 and 1878, Senn studied medicine at the University of Munich, Germany, and returned to Milwaukee to practice. He became a superb teacher and a respected clinician. J. B. Murphy described Senn in much the way others described Martin: "His industry, zeal and perseverance were recognized qualities."[2] Murphy said of Senn that he did things now and in the present. He performed systematic and original experiments with animals and his presentations

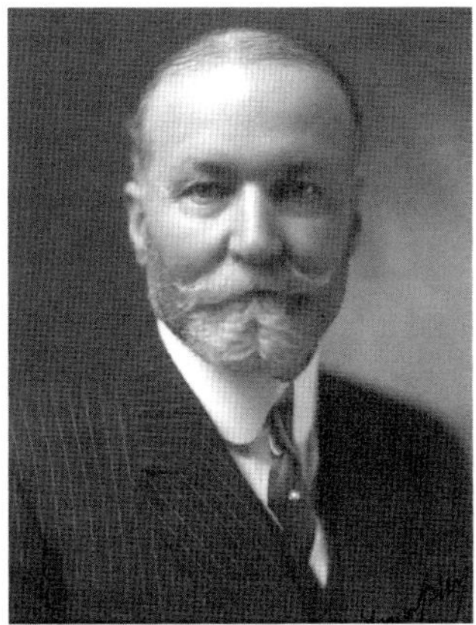

17.1. Dr. John B. Murphy, celebrated Chicago surgeon.

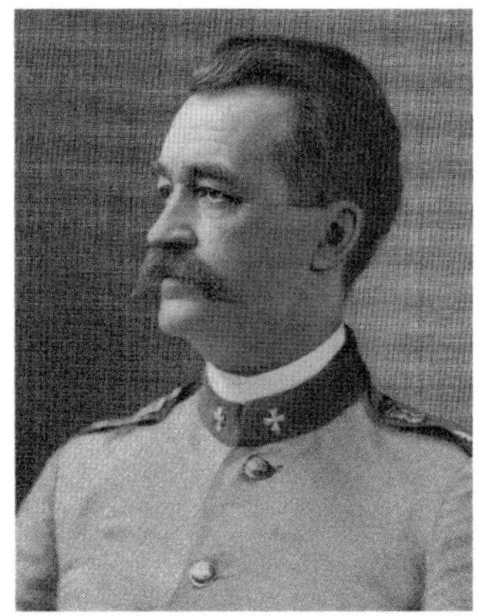

17.2. Dr. Nicholas Senn, renowned clinical instructor and surgical researcher.

contained his data and original observations. He became president of the American Medical Association and served many other surgical organizations. Senn's contributions to the practice of surgery included numerous publications and 27 major textbooks.[2]

DR. ALBERT J. OCHSNER

Albert Ochsner (Figure 17.3) was born in 1858 in Baraboo, WI, and grew up on his family's farm. During his formative years, he helped on the farm for seven months of the year and attended school for five months during the winter. Ochsner, too, passed the county teacher's examination and taught school for five winter terms. He went on to receive a bachelor's degree with honors from the University of Wisconsin and received his medical degree from Rush Medical College in 1886. During the next two-and-a-half years, Ochsner completed an internship at Presbyterian Hospital in Chicago and studied extensively at several famous clinics in Europe. Upon his return to Chicago, he rose rapidly in the ranks until at age 42 he became chair of clinical surgery at the University of Illinois. Ochsner was respected as a great teacher and authored numerous publications and multiple textbooks. His work on the conservative treatment of appendicitis, although controversial, demonstrated his clinical and diagnostic acumen. His mentoring of his cousin Alton

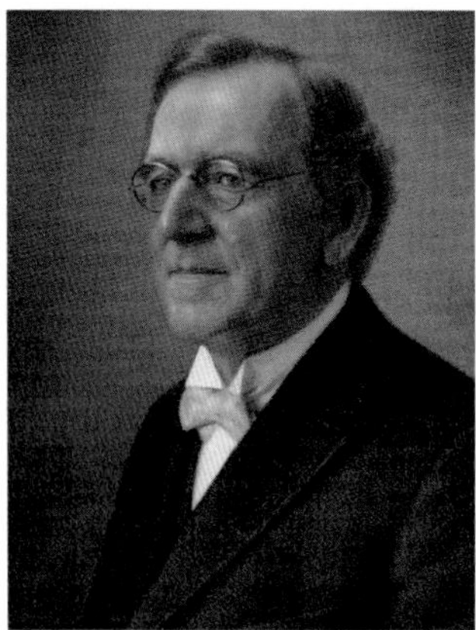

17.3. Dr. Albert J. Ochsner, one of the founders of the ACS and ACS President, 1923 to 1924.

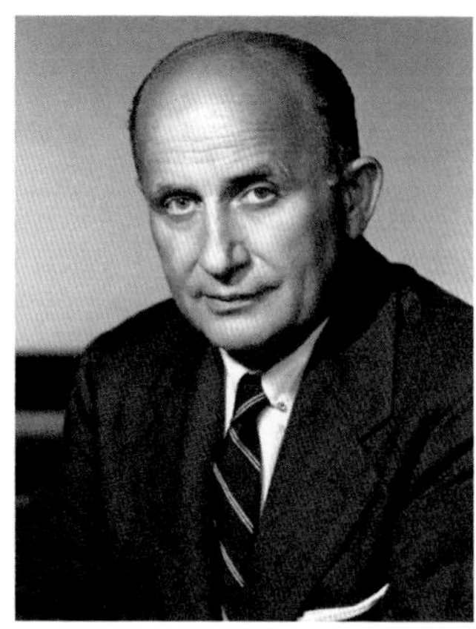

17.4. Dr. Robert M. Zollinger, chair of surgery, The Ohio State University, 1947 to 1974; ACS President, 1961 to 1962.

Ochsner significantly guided the latter's medical training and made it feasible for him to help found the Ochsner Clinic in New Orleans.[3]

Dr. Robert M. Zollinger

Robert Zollinger (Figure 17.4) was born in 1903 on the family farm in Millersport, OH. When he was not in school, Zollinger performed chores from sunrise to sunset. During the school term he was expected to perform chores after school and before completing his homework. It was important to Zollinger's parents that he receive a good education, as they had not had that opportunity. When Robert was in his early teens, his father purchased a pony and buggy and arranged for him to deliver milk and cream to vacationers in cottages on a local lake. His parents insisted that he approach the deliveries responsibly and treat them as a serious business. Robert said, "This project taught me a lot about human nature and how to deal with the public—and how to get the bottles back!"[4]

Even after Zollinger began attending The Ohio State University, Columbus, his father insisted that he return home on weekends to work on the farm. His weekend farm chores kept him so busy that he had little time to study. He said of the impact of his work on the farm on weekends, "It's a wonder I could pass because I spent a lot of time shelling corn for the pigs and doing other farm work. This left me with no college social life at all. It was a pretty miserable first year."[4]

Finding funds to pay his tuition was a constant struggle until his third year of medical school, when he took a job in the pharmacy of a nearby institute, where he stayed employed until he graduated from medical school two years later. After an internship at Peter Bent Brigham Hospital in Boston, Zollinger completed his residency at Western Reserve University, Cleveland, OH. He was appointed chief resident at Western Reserve, but after six weeks he resigned to return with his chief, Dr. Elliott Cutler, to Peter Bent Brigham Hospital, where he was again appointed chief resident and, two years later, became a junior member of the surgical staff. Following more than three years in the Army in World War II, Zollinger returned to Boston, but by April 1946 he moved to The Ohio State University department of surgery; a few months later, he became chairman. He developed a stellar surgery department, with one of the premier surgery training programs in the country. His accomplishments were many and varied, but he most often is remembered for describing Zollinger-Ellison Syndrome. As Martin had experienced, some colleagues made fun of Zollinger's rural upbringing, but, unlike Martin, he appeared unmoved.[4]

DR. WARREN H. COLE

Warren Cole (Figure 17.5) was born in 1898 on the family farm in Clay County, KS. When he was five years old, his mother died after undergoing a hysterectomy for vaginal bleeding. Her untimely death was one of the reasons Cole decided to become a surgeon. The hardships of growing up on a frontier farm were increased without a mother to run the household. At age seven or eight, Cole became the family cook whenever the housekeeper was unavailable.

Of his rural upbringing Cole said,

> I consider myself extremely fortunate to have been born and raised on the farm.... There are numerous advantages in this life which cannot be equalled by living in the city. Life on the farm and going to a country school were, in my estimation, very

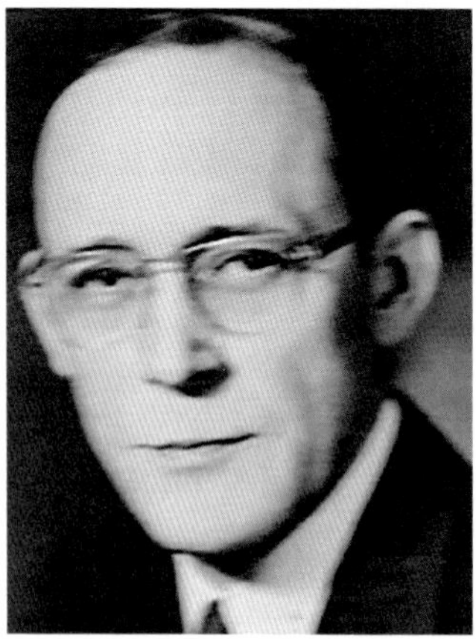

17.5. Dr. Warren H. Cole, chair of surgery, University of Illinois College of Medicine in Chicago, 1936 to 1966; ACS President, 1955 to 1956.

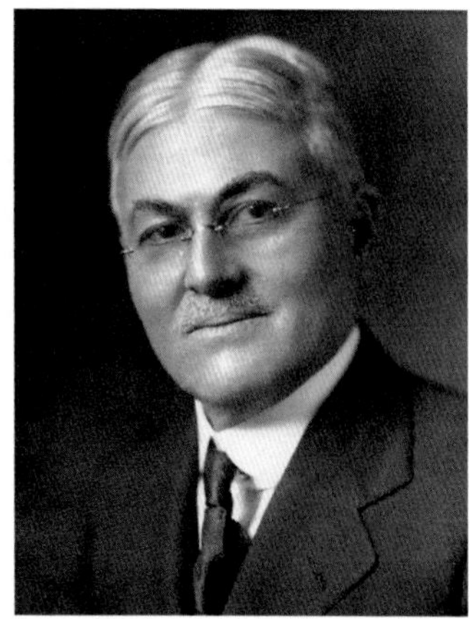

17.6. Dr. George W. Crile, one of the founders of the Cleveland Clinic, in 1921; ACS President, 1916 to 1917.

> advantageous to my future, largely because of the many character-building hardships we had to undergo. In my opinion, these hardships develop character, that is, tolerance, patience, willingness to work hard and many other desirable characteristics.[5]

In summation, he said, "I am saying that I was not a spoiled brat, which is the kind of character some youngsters develop who live in the city and have all material things they want."[5]

Cole and his brothers performed most of the farm labor except during harvest, when farmhands were brought in to help. He agreed with Martin that the most difficult task was shocking the wheat: standing the bundled wheat on end and covering it with additional wheat to keep it dry. Like Martin, Cole described this work as interminable and fatiguing and said, "The discipline needed to perform such work surely built character."[5] These experiences developed in Cole a capacity for hard work over long hours, an aptitude for keen observation, and an appreciation of the importance of work, family, and education. Cole was convinced that growing up on a farm built his character and made it possible for him to become a successful surgeon and researcher.[5]

Dr. George W. Crile

George Crile (Figure 17.6), another successful surgeon, was born in 1864 on his family's farm in Chili, OH. Crile and his siblings also worked long hours during the harvest season. Crile's father gave each of his children a lamb, calf, or pig to care for as an incentive to work and to teach his children thrift. He gave each of his children a colt for their 16th birthday with the same expectations. Crile said of this experience,

> It tied each one of the children to the others and made us personally concerned with the success of the farm, for since each of the eight at various times actually owned sheep, cattle and horses, there was no lack of interest in the welfare of the stock. I cannot conceive of a better method to induce development of character, incentive in work and habits of thrift, and at the same time give means for substantial financial help."[6]

Crile said, "[M]y father's farm was a valuable laboratory. In many ways Father was ahead of his times. He had a very inquiring and logical mind. Empirically he was a scientific farmer...." Growing up on a farm, Crile believed he learned firsthand about the laws of heredity, the intelligence of both domestic and wild animals, and the impact of domestication on farm animals. In summary of his rural upbringing, Crile said,

> It was some years before I realized the advantages of a childhood on the farm, but now I know that I was fortunate. If a lad learns early the rudiments of thinking, if he comprehends the sequence of cause and effect, the ability to learn to reason in the abstract is not a difficult step.[6]

Of his many accomplishments, cofounding the prestigious Cleveland Clinic best exemplifies his ability to develop and organize such a major institution.[6]

Drs. Charles and William Mayo

Probably the most famous exemplars of the impact of a farm childhood on a surgical career are Charles and William Mayo (Figure 17.7).

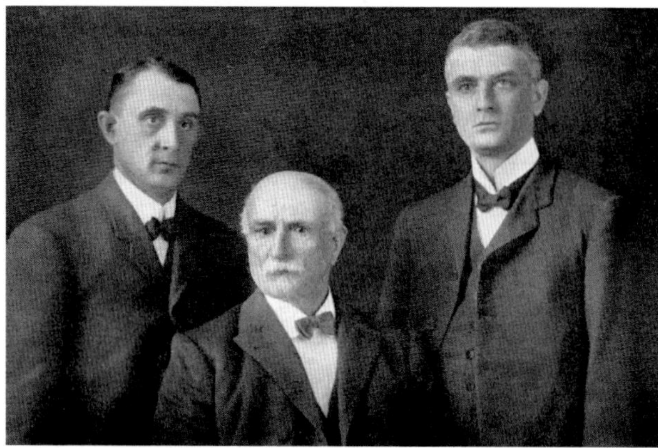

17.7. The Mayo Brothers, founders of the Mayo Clinic, with their father. From left: Charles H. Mayo, William Worrall Mayo, and William James Mayo. Both younger Mayos became ACS Presidents.

William was born in 1861 in Le Sueur, MN, and his brother Charles in 1865 in Rochester, MN. Even when young, the brothers were expected to perform chores on the family farm. They drove the cows out in the morning and back in at night, cared for the family garden, brought water from the well, and kept the wood box filled. They also cared for their doctor father's horses, cleaned his office, and drove him on his patient rounds. Their father did not want his sons to be idle. Most certainly he instilled strong character traits in his sons that substantially contributed to their notable careers and their creation of the Mayo Clinic.[7]

Dr. Earl Mayne

Earl Mayne (Figure 17.8) was born in 1866 in Mason City, IA—the youngest of eight children on a small family farm. His parents provided a sturdy environment for their large family. By working on the family farm, Mayne said, he "learned the value of industry, self-reliance, and self-respect."[8] He raised cattle to help finance his undergraduate studies in civil engineering at the University of Iowa, Iowa City. He described waiting tables and cutting firewood so he could pay for a hired hand to do his share of the farm labor. His civil engineering train-

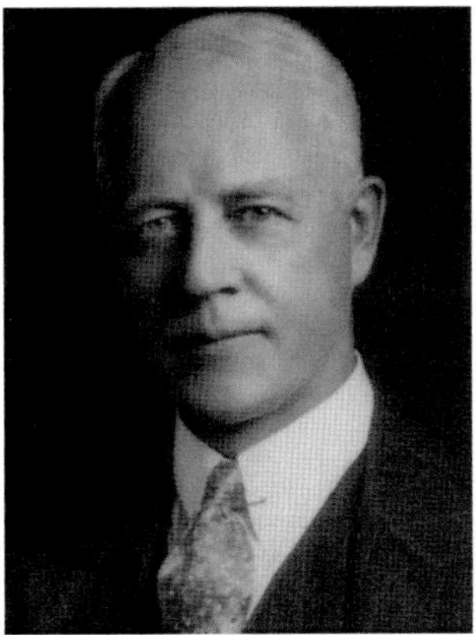

17.8. Dr. Earl Mayne, charter member of the ACS and member of the ACS Board of Governors.

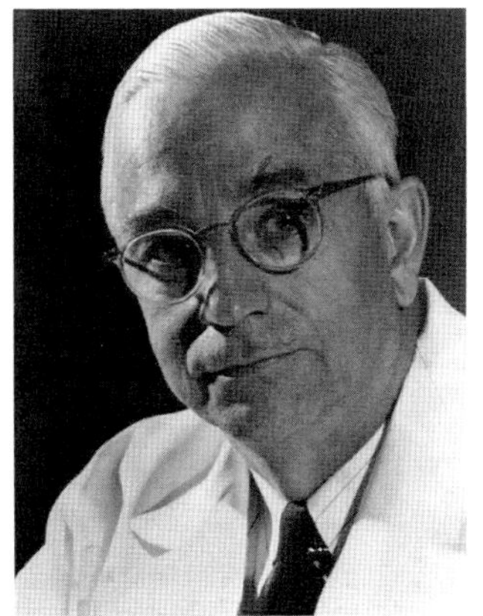

17.9. Dr. Owen H. Wangensteen, chair of surgery, University of Minnesota, 1930 to 1967; ACS President, 1959 to 1960.

ing enabled him to secure a position as a bridge builder and to earn money to attend Bellevue Hospital Medical College in New York. He then practiced medicine in Brooklyn, NY. He worked hard to establish his medical practice, which grew rapidly, and he became a successful and well-known surgeon.[8]

Dr. Owen H. Wangensteen

Owen Wangensteen (Figure 17.9) was born in 1898 in Lake Park, MN. When he was seven years old, his mother died and his father raised Owen, his brothers, and his sister. Although his father stressed to his children the importance of an education, they also were expected to participate in the farm chores. Owen believed he contributed more to running the farm than his brothers and is quoted as saying, "They learned to hunt, but I learned to work. And I think I got the best of the deal."[9] An example of his dedication to the farm work was that when the family herd of sows could not farrow their young, he spent three weeks delivering 300 piglets and, in the process, saved the herd. He graduated from the University of Minnesota Medical School, Minneapolis, in 1922. In 1931, at age 32, he became chair of surgery at the University of Minnesota and developed one of the greatest surgical research centers in the world. Both his research and clinical work were marked by innovation and resulted in 38 graduates of his residency becoming chairs of departments of surgery, a legacy that few surgeons can claim.[9]

As these prominent men demonstrate, Franklin Martin was not the only surgeon who benefited from a rural upbringing. Their rural backgrounds also had an impact on their leadership abilities, their character, and their self-confidence.

Not only surgeons believe they benefited from a rural/farm upbringing. Following are just a few examples of nonsurgeons who are eloquent on the subject.

Beuna Coburn Carlson

Beuna Coburn Carlson wrote very eloquently in her book, *Farm Girl*, about farm life in western Wisconsin during the Dust Bowl and the Great Depression. She said of the people who survived the adversity of these times,

> Not only surviving adversity, but also prevailing over misfortune with humor, love, a sense of beauty, many of these farmers and their children went on to become leaders in the 1940s, during World War II, and beyond. The hope, the can-do spirit, and the determination not to give up were the principles that produced a generation of strong, determined, innovative women and men.[10]

She describes with great love and affection that her parents taught her and her siblings that bitterness and hopelessness were not the way to deal with adversity. Rather it was to find happiness, joy, and pleasure in the multitude of small successes that occurred frequently on a farm.[10] She was guided by these teachings throughout her life and they served her well.

Dr. Maurice Hilleman

Maurice Hilleman was born in 1919 and grew up in Depression-era poverty in the harsh plains of southeastern Montana.[11] His mother died two days after he was born and his father, at his mother's request, gave Maurice over to be raised by an aunt and uncle.[12] Hilleman describes raising and selling numerous vegetables, chickens, eggs, and flowers. He also was responsible for caring for the horses and chickens. The summers were very hot and the winters freezing. Life was brutal.[13]

After completing his graduate studies at the University of Chicago, Hilleman went into industry and develop vaccines for measles, mumps, rubella (German measles), chickenpox, hepatitis A, hepatitis B, pneumococcus, meningococcus, and Haemophilus influenza type B, and in the process likely saved more lives than all other scientists combined.[11] He was bold and forward thinking and, like Martin, when he saw that something needed to be accomplished, he proceeded. Dr. Paul Offit says in his book about Hilleman that he used a committee-of-one approach when making decisions, an approach not unlike Martin's and one that was successful for him, too.[14] Offit also said, "Hilleman didn't see his career as improbable, reasoning that his farming background was perfect training for a scientist to create life-saving vaccines."[15] Hilleman himself said of his farm upbringing, "When you're brought up on a farm, you have a lot of general knowledge."[15] His five surviving brothers also were successful in professions as wide-ranging as anatomy and physiology to airplane design. Although his brothers were highly accomplished, as described by Offit, "Maurice's relentless, unending drive was unique."[15]

REFERENCES

1. Davis, L. (1938). *J.B. Murphy: Stormy Petrel of Surgery* (pp. 3-57). New York, NY: G. P. Putnam's Sons.
2. Murphy, J. B. (1908). Nicholas Senn, Ph. D., M. D., LL. D. *Surg Gynecol & Obstet,* VI(2), 116-120.
3. Ventura, H. O. (2001). Albert Ochsner, MD: Chicago surgeon and mentor to Alton Ochsner. *Ochsner J,* 3(4), 223-225.
4. Miller, C. A. (2014). *The Big Z: The Life of Robert M. Zollinger, MD* (pp. 7-184). Chicago, IL: American College of Surgeons.
5. Connaughton, D. (1991). *Warren Cole, MD, and the Ascent of Scientific Surgery* (pp. 1-32). Champaign, IL: University of Illinois Press.
6. Crile, G., editor (1947). *George Crile: An Autobiography,* vol. 1 (pp. 3–22). Phila-

delphia, PA, and New York, NY: J. B. Lippincott Company.

7. Clapesattle, H. (1941). *The Doctors Mayo* (pp. 168-170). Minneapolis, MN: University of Minnesota Press.
8. Klein, S. B., Sasser, W. F. (2015). The Mayne legacy: A look back at an influential charter member of the ACS. *Bull Am Coll Surg*, 100(9), 18-21.
9. Buchwald, H. (2020). *Surgical Renaissance in the Heartland: A Memoir of the Wangensteen Era* (pp. 17-18). Minneapolis, MN: University of Minnesota Press.
10. Carlson, B. C. (2020). *Farm Girl* (p. xii). Madison, WI: The University of Wisconsin Press.
11. Offit, P. A. (2007). *Vaccinated* (pp. xi-xii). New York, NY: HarperCollins Publishers, Inc.
12. Ibid., p. 4.
13. Ibid., pp. 5-6.
14. Ibid., p. 17.
15. Ibid., pp. 186-187.

ACKNOWLEDGMENTS

I need to acknowledge many people for their assistance with this book. First, I must acknowledge and thank Susan Rishworth, former Archivist for the American College of Surgeons (ACS), for encouraging me to take on the project of researching Dr. Franklin Martin's early years in Wisconsin and for supporting me over the years as I carried out the project. Although it was slow going at first, she always was confident that I would eventually complete the project.

The superb editing of Tina Woelke of the ACS Division of Integrated Communications was instrumental in facilitating the creation of a quality manuscript. She read and edited the multiple editions of every chapter and helped convert my at times faulty prose into more elegant phraseology. Her enthusiasm for the enterprise encouraged and inspired me when I most needed it. She was willing and able to assist me with every aspect of producing this book. She was indispensable in my quest to produce a worthwhile book. Lynn Kahn, then Director of the ACS Division of Integrated Communications, was instrumental in getting the book project up and going. I am grateful to Kira Plotts and Sue Kawecki, who proofread the book. The exceptional editorial skills of Diane Schneidman of the same division at the ACS were exceedingly helpful as I completed the final manuscript.

I must thank Don Nakayama, MD, FACS; Kenneth Davis, PhD; Carol Scott-Conner, MD, FACS; Ms. Rishworth; and David Nahrwold, MD, FACS, for critiquing the early chapters and getting me on the right track. I must thank my wife, Susan Walgenbach Telford, PhD, who often listened to my thoughts about Martin and joined me frequently as I visited sites and researched his life in Wisconsin. She was my touchstone; if I could convince her of my latest theory about the impact of his early life on Martin's phenomenally successful career, then I knew I was headed in the right direction. It was wonderful to have someone close who would get just as excited as I did when I discovered something new and interesting about Martin's early life.

Without the assistance of the ACS Archivists, past and present, I would not have been able to navigate my way through the 90 boxes of the Martin papers and other materials in the ACS Archives. They skillfully located documents in advance of my many visits to the Archives, and expertly and accurately copied untold numbers of documents, journal articles, and book chapters. The present Archivist, Meghan Kennedy, and the Assistant Archivist, Michael Beesley, have been especially helpful in locating materials. The previous Archivist, Adam Carey, also was of great assistance.

Numerous people and organizations in the Oconomowoc, Ixonia, Watertown, and Elroy areas of Wisconsin helped me as I investigated Martin and his ties to the area. The Oconomowoc Area Historical Society and the Dodge/Jefferson Counties Genealogical Society libraries both were excellent resources and their society members and staff were of tremendous assistance. Both organizations invited me to present the results of my early research to their societies, which led to new clues from the audience. At one presentation, I met the granddaughter of Martin's cousin Washington Fulmer. Mary Waarvik of the Elroy Historical Society was helpful with information about the Elroy Seminary that Martin attended.

Because my son Andrew is buried in La Belle Cemetery in Oconomowoc, WI, where many members of the Martin family and their descendants are buried, I was asked to become a member of the Board of Trustees of the Cemetery Association and later president of the board. With the help of our sextant, Steve Tucker, I was able to identify the burial sites and review the records of those members of the Martin family buried in the cemetery. Using this information and the dates on the individual monuments, I was able to verify information I had from other sources and in some cases establish new information about the Martin family. I also was able to review the Carlin family records in Oak Hill Cemetery in Watertown, WI. When conducting genealogical and historical research, especially when looking back 150 years and more, cemetery records and grave markers can be the only easily accessible source of information about families and can lead to other sources.

All the families who are the present owners of houses that had been previously owned by members of the extended Martin and Carlin families welcomed me into their homes and were enormously helpful and open to my requests for information. They all became interested in the project. Especially helpful were Tim and Rose Burns, who own William Fulmer's home. They generously gave me several of the bricks from the Fulmer brickyard that were on their property. Also helpful were Pam and Harold Coppernoll and Richard and Heidi Hogan. Tom and Sandy Zillmer had in their possession extensive Fulmer family records and generously shared them with me. Sadly, Tom and Sandy died before they could see my completed work. Rebecca Eash gave generously of her time, helping me locate information and teaching me how to complete this type of research. Many members of the Dodge/Jefferson Counties Genealogical Society and the Oconomowoc Historical Society were particularly helpful.

Finally, I must thank David B. Hoyt, MD, FACS, ACS Executive Director, for supporting my work and for his willingness to publish the manuscript.

Illustration Credits

Frontispiece

Franklin H. Martin, MD, FACS, Founder of the American College of Surgeons, circa 1900. *Franklin Martin Collection, Archives of the American College of Surgeons.*

Chapter Pages Background Art

Pages from Franklin Martin's handwritten first draft of his 1933 autobiography, *The Joy of Living. Franklin Martin Collection, Archives of the American College of Surgeons.*

Chapter 1

1.1. Edmond Martin, Franklin's father. *Franklin Martin Collection, Archives of the American College of Surgeons.*

1.2. William and Caroline (Phelps) Martin, Franklin's paternal grandparents. *Oconomowoc Historical Society.*

1.3. Josephine Carlin Martin, Franklin's mother. *Franklin Martin Collection, Archives of the American College of Surgeons.*

1.4. 1862 plat map of Ixonia Township showing the location of the Martin and Carlin homesteads and the location of Martin's Uncle Luther Hatch's and his stepfather Elon Munger's family homesteads. *Public document.*

1.5. Recent photograph of the Carlin family's home in Ixonia Township. The site of this home agrees with the site identified on plat maps from the mid-1800s. In addition, close examination of the foundation of the home reveals that it was constructed with fieldstone, making it likely that the home was built in the

CHAPTER 2

CHAPTER 3

3.1. Uncle Adolphus Guilder, Franklin's mentor when he worked in the flour mill. *Franklin Martin Collection, Archives of the American College of Surgeons.*

3.2. Uncle George Fulmer, owner of the Fulmer brickyard. *Oconomowoc Historical Society.*

3.3. Fulmer brickyard crew. From left: Franklin Martin, Julius Besendorf, Thomas Fulmer, Richard Fulmer, and Washington Fulmer. The three Fulmers were Franklin's cousins. *Personal collection of Donald Zillmer.*

3.4. Brick from the Fulmer brickyard. Gift from Tim and Rose Burns, who now own Martin's Uncle William Fulmer's home where the bricks were found. The color and style of the brick are consistent with the type of bricks made in the Fulmer brickyard. *Author's collection.*

3.5. Flanagan Building in downtown Oconomowoc, WI, which was constructed with Fulmer brick. The building is unusual because of its arched brick window casings. The Fulmer brickyard was the only local brickyard where beveled brick molds were used to make the bricks necessary to construct arched window casings. *Author's collection.*

CHAPTER 4

4.1. Field where Franklin was binding oats when he saw Dr. Daniel McLaren Miller drive by in his buggy. *Author's collection.*

4.2. Aunt Mary Carlin, Martin's supportive maternal aunt. *Franklin Martin Collection, Archives of the American College of Surgeons.*

4.3. Watertown Bank Building in the late 1800s. Dr. William Spalding's office, where Franklin apprenticed, was on the second floor. *Dodge/Jefferson Counties Genealogical Society.*

4.4. Grandmother Caroline Martin. *Oconomowoc Historical Society.*

4.5. Branch Road in Ixonia today, where it traverses what was the Martin homestead. *Author's collection.*

4.6. Dr. Nicholas Senn, another famous Chicago surgeon from Wisconsin. *Franklin Martin Collection, Archives of the American College of Surgeons.*

CHAPTER 5

5.1. Franklin Martin, circa the time he left for medical school in Chicago. *Franklin Martin Collection, Archives of the American College of Surgeons.*

5.2. Chicago Medical College (26th Street and Prairie Avenue) circa 1880, when Martin was a student. *Courtesy of Galter Health Sciences Library & Learning Center, Northwestern University Feinberg School of Medicine, Chicago, IL, USA.*

5.3. Uncle Addison Carlin, Martin's supportive uncle who assisted him financially during medical school. *Franklin Martin Collection, Archives of the American College of Surgeons.*

5.4. Oak Grove School, Oak Grove, WI, where Martin taught. *Franklin Martin Collection, Archives of the American College of Surgeons.*

5.5. Recent photograph of the Silver Lake area, where Martin's mother Josephine, his stepfather Elon Munger, and sister Jeanette lived in the 1870s and 1880s and where Martin spent a month relaxing before returning to Chicago to begin his internship. *Author's collection.*

5.6. Mercy Hospital (26th Street and Calumet Avenue) circa 1880, when Martin did his internship. *Courtesy of Galter Health Sciences Library & Learning Center, Northwestern University Feinberg School of Medicine, Chicago, IL, USA.*

Chapter 6

6.1. Central Hall Building (22nd Street and Wabash Avenue), where Martin had his first office, late 1800s. *Franklin Martin Collection, Archives of the American College of Surgeons.*

6.2. Chicago South-Side Medico-Social Society members. Martin is third from the right in the middle row. Lorenzo Potter is third from the left in the middle row. Edmund Doering, President of the Society, is fourth from the left in the middle row. *Franklin Martin Collection, Archives of the American College of Surgeons.*

Chapter 7

7.1. Isabelle Hollister Martin (left) and Franklin Martin (right) at about the time of their marriage. *Franklin Martin Collection, Archives of the American College of Surgeons.*

7.2. Martin golfing with friends. In the first photograph (a) he is on the left-hand side and Isabelle is preparing to hit the ball. In (b) he is second from the left. *Franklin Martin Collection, Archives of the American College of Surgeons.*

Chapter 9

9.1. Drs. William J. (left) and Charles H. (right) Mayo. *Used with permission of Mayo Foundation for Medical Education and Research. All rights reserved.*

CHAPTER 10

10.1. Advertisement in the *Journal of the American Medical Association* for the Post-Graduate Medical School of Chicago, which Martin had a prominent part in organizing. *From the* Journal of the American Medical Association, 1889. *Author's collection.*

CHAPTER 11

11.1. Dr. Martin's official ACS portrait from the 1920s. *Franklin Martin Collection, Archives of the American College of Surgeons.*

11.2. Dr. John B. Murphy, another famous Chicago surgeon raised in rural Wisconsin. *Franklin Martin Collection, Archives of the American College of Surgeons.*

11.3. The four young surgeons who assisted in the initial planning for the publication of *Surgery, Gynecology & Obstetrics* (clockwise from top left): Frederic A. Besley, Allen B. Kanavel, William R. Cubbins, and John Hollister. *Franklin Martin Collection, Archives of the American College of Surgeons.*

11.4. Volume 1, Number 1, of *Surgery, Gynecology & Obstetrics.* Note the number of prominent surgeons listed on the editorial staff and as contributors. *Franklin Martin Collection, Archives of the American College of Surgeons.*

11.5. Original Board of Regents of the American College of Surgeons. *Franklin Martin Collection, Archives of the American College of Surgeons.*

CHAPTER 13

13.1. Dr. Frank Simpson. *Franklin Martin Collection, Archives of the American College of Surgeons.*

13.2. Members of the Advisory Commission of the Council of National Defense. *Franklin Martin Collection, Archives of the American College of Surgeons.*

13.3. Members of the Council of National Defense and the Advisory Commission. Seated, from left: David F. Houston, Josephus Daniels, Newton D. Baker (Chairman), Franklin K. Lane, and William Wilson. Standing, from left: Grosvenor Clarkson (Secretary), Julius Rosenwald, Bernard Baruch, Daniel Willard, Franklin H. Martin, Hollis Godfrey, Howard Coffin, and Walter Gifford. *Franklin Martin Collection, Archives of the American College of Surgeons.*

13.4. Martin in his Army uniform. *Franklin Martin Collection, Archives of the American College of Surgeons.*

Chapter 14

Chapter 15

Chapter 16

Chapter 17

17.4. Dr. Robert M. Zollinger, chair of surgery, The Ohio State University, 1947 to 1974; ACS President, 1961 to 1962. *Franklin Martin Collection, Archives of the American College of Surgeons.*
17.5. Dr. Warren H. Cole, chair of surgery, University of Illinois College of Medicine in Chicago, 1936 to 1966; ACS President, 1955 to 1956. *Franklin Martin Collection, Archives of the American College of Surgeons.*
17.6. Dr. George Crile, one of the founders of the Cleveland Clinic, in 1921; ACS President, 1916 to 1917. *Franklin Martin Collection, Archives of the American College of Surgeons.*
17.7 The Mayo Brothers, founders of the Mayo Clinic, with their father. From left: Charles H. Mayo, William Worrall Mayo, and William James Mayo. Both younger Mayos became ACS Presidents. *Franklin Martin Collection, Archives of the American College of Surgeons.*
17.8. Dr. Earl Mayne, charter member of the ACS and member of the ACS Board of Governors. *Archives of the American College of Surgeons.*
17.9. Dr. Owen H. Wangensteen, chair of surgery, University of Minnesota, 1930 to 1967; ACS President, 1959 to 1960. *Archives of the American College of Surgeons.*

NOTE

The author, editor, and publisher gratefully acknowledge the permission granted to reproduce the copyright material in this book.

Every effort has been made to trace copyright holders and to obtain their permission for the use of copyright material. The publisher apologizes for any errors or omissions in the above list and would be grateful if notified of any corrections that should be incorporated in future reprints or editions of this book.

Index

Page locators in *italics* indicate photographs and illustrations.